SACRED BIRTH POWER MAI
Intuitive Birthing

This book was first published in 2013 entitled Manifest Sacred Birth, Intuitive Birthing Techniques by Ishtara Blue. This is the revised second edition 2022.

Intuitive Birthing was a term coined by Ishtara Rose when she first started to write this book between 2007 and 2009 whilst preparing for and birthing 2 babies during that time. Ishtara then gathered together her personal notes and self published them in 2013. Now due to popular demand she has revised and updated the material.

Intuitive Birthing is the core essence of sacred birth and the message that Ishtara is passionate about sharing. This is not about right and wrong ways of birthing, but finding clear and easy alignment to your intuition to birth how it is right for YOU to birth. And we are all unique.

By following the intuitive birthing techniques in this book, and finding your sacred birth power mantras, you can birth clearly connected and tuned in to follow your unique body clear signals and clear intuition, so that your birth can be blissful and even pain free.

If a birthing womb-an is in a 'sacred' place, she hears her intuition easily so she can open her light womb up wide. When she cannot hear the inner voice, she acts from a place of fear, she is 'scared'. It is this fear which blocks the birth hormones from being released and prevents her from opening up her womb easily and without pain.

In PART 1 SACRED BIRTH POWER MANTRAS Ishtara shares ten easy steps to finding your own Sacred Birth Power Mantras. In this process you will find your own core mantras from your own subconscious, whilst directly addressing any birthing fears from within, to manifest your dream sacred birth intention in beautiful flow.

In PART 2 INTUITIVE BIRTHING TECHNIQUES reflect on key intuitive birthing techniques to bring you into clarity, including such things as visualisation, meditation, prayer, ceremony and more. These are designed for regular practise from around week twenty of the pregnancy, but to familiarise yourself with from before that time, then to use during the actual birth itself.

In PART 3 BIRTH MANIFESTATION bring it all together to create your own birth manifestation programme

The techniques in this book are ones that Ishtara draws upon in her healing and priestess mystery school training. They can also be applied for many other birthing and pregnancy issues such as resolving conception difficulties, releasing, healing and forgiving past birth trauma, or using them to connect to your intuition as a parent.

Acknowledgements 2009

I am eternally grateful for 'Joanna Josephina May' for guidance and inspiration, who brought me the messages and got the book written. A big thank you to my children for their creativity, magical spark, and inspiration and to Matthew for positive encouragement and safely holding the space when I birthed our children. Thank you to the wonderful girls who have come and taken my children off for walks so I can write - Victoria, Kes, Anna and Moon; to all those friends, teachers and therapists who supported and inspired me when I was pregnant and during the births; and course thank you to my extended family for your ongoing love, help and support.

Acknowledgements, Revised edition 2022

It first must be said that all I do and write comes from my spirit guides and team who I constantly work closely with. I am exceptionally grateful every day to be blessed to find myself in a place where I am able to be channel for and with them, to hear them and to open to the Light that is forth coming at this time.

I wish also to take opportunity to thank 'my' online light worker community of women, you know who you are, those incredible women who inspire - I am in honour and deepest respect for the women (and men) who courageously take time to 'face their stuff' and go deep to step up and speak up at this time. I also wish to express my immense respect for all the priestesses who have opened their hearts on my courses, who are my own teachers, and to the High Priestesses Bridget, Emma, Kathy, Dawn.

I would not be here doing what I do, if it was not for Margaret Hunt, my own priestess teacher who guided me through much during my own deep long dark night of the soul commencing in and around 2017.

I must acknowledge my children who of course are the ones who led to the book in the first place, and who unknowingly and sometimes unwillingly (!) support my dedicated ongoing spiritual work. They have been with me every step of the way, and patiently put up with 'my unusual ways', whilst I am constantly taught new things by their 'unusual ways', their bright intelligence and spark, as they courageously carve out their own pathways as they grow in unknown pastures during this new age, often surprising us all into unexpected situations.

Thank you must also go to Florian, a bright light, who is able to go deeper to the underlying truths and energy, a gift indeed.

For my beautiful children
My gratitude and divinely infinite love for you
May you be forever blessed.

For all birthing women, men, children and babies
May your births be blessed and beautiful.

For Mother Mary, Mary Magdalene and the Queen of Heaven
Divine Mother
Queen of Angels
Goddess of Light

For the Divine Mother within us all
To help birthing women and men all over the world
To birth in peace, in love
To return to their Goddess power
 Whilst giving life.

For all
For the highest good of all
For Light, For Love

When You Have a Dream

Follow its Light

Birth in the Light

May all Women Return to the Light

It is from Light Women bring Life unto Fruition

From Light Life Is Borne

Preface

I am not a professional birth specialist, but I do know that you can create your own birth to be as beautiful as you can imagine, because I have done it twice myself and have seen many others do it by using these methods.

When I became pregnant for the first time, I put all my knowledge of meditation and holistic therapies into practise, and designed this programme for myself in order to have my beautiful sacred birth. When I became pregnant again, I put the same methods to use and after another beautiful birth, I realised it really does work. People would say how lucky I was to have had two wonderful births, but it was not luck. I consciously did the work to create it to be like that by taking time every day to fill with Light and intention and clear out all the blocks in the various ways outlined in this book. I even managed to turn my birth around when it seemed to be heading off in the 'wrong' direction, using these techniques.

Why *Intuitive Birth*? Why *Sacred Birth*? To birth well, you need to be turned within. In this way you are birthing in a' trance state', in touch with your instincts. Intuition is the way to hear your "Higher Self", to be in a sacred place. There is no right or wrong way to birth, only what is appropriate for you and your baby; you are unique and your situation is unique.

This method then is about creating the internal and external space to tune into your intuition clearly for your Sacred Birth. It is not saying it is 'sacred' and 'right' to have a home birth and 'wrong' and 'not sacred' to birth in hospital; but I do share that to birth in hospital with intervention could make it more difficult to hear your intuition clearly. However, in the event that your intuition says "go to hospital", then that is what is right for you and the book gives tips on how to maintain your sacred space anywhere, as well as to help to decipher between fear and instinct.

In order to birth from your intuition, you need to have worked on releasing any internal blocks and targeting any hidden trauma, so that you are completely relaxed, knowing that whatever you feel internally could emerge in your birth, and if anything does arise during birth then you feel comfortable to turn it around with techniques to quickly do so. Using manifestation techniques alongside intuitive birth techniques is the basis of this programme. The power of words, visualisation and ceremony will enable you to manifest all that is within your heart. However this is not just manifestation through positive affirmation, but you will go into the subconscious to actually target any trauma and find your very own personal mantras directly from your own inner psyche. The world is your mirror. Whatever you ask for will happen for you if you believe it will and want it to, and if you have released any issues that stop you from believing it. Energy follows thought and emotion. So we work first and foremost with the energy within all things.

The programme in this book will therefore help you to discover and heal any blocks to become a clear channel. For example, by following this programme you may discover that you want a pain-free birth but inside there is some resistance that makes you believe that this is not possible. You will, therefore, use the techniques within this programme to find and release this resistance so that you can fully know it is fully possible - at the very root. From this belief you can go on to enjoy a happy, pain-free birth.

Happy Birthing! May your womb be filled with Light!

Book Contents

Introduction
Manifestation, Intuition and The World as your Mirror.

Part One - Create Your Own Birthing Mantras
Create your personal birthing power mantras in ten easy steps.

Part Two - Intuitive Birthing
Intuitive Birthing Techniques to fill up with womb light.

Clear Thought
Clear Emotion
Clear Body
Clear Spirit
Clear Connection
Clear Birth
Clear Parent

Part Three - Birth Manifestation
The Birth Manifestation Programme, from approximately week 32

Appendix
Examples of supporting evidence
Bibliography

Exercise Contents

Part One - Create your Birth Power Mantras

Part Two - Intuitive Birthing Techniques

1 Clear Thoughts

2 Clear Emotions

3 Clear Body

4 Clear Spirit

Exercise to Invoke Rays of Light
Visualisation for Angelic Healing
Clear Channel of Light Meditation
The Birth Manifestation Ceremony
Visualisation for Sacred Space

5 Clear Connection
Temple of Power Visualisation
Invocation for your Ancient Midwife
Examples of Relationship Mantras
Attracting Love Meditation
Loving Eyes Meditation
Male and Female Within Visualisation
Healing your Relationship with the Perineum Massage
Full Power Self meditation
Conscious Communication

6 Clear Birth
The Birth Rehearsal
The Birth Reminder card
The Birth Plan
Natural Pain Management in Stage One
Birth Calming Checklist for an Anxious Mother
Birth Calming Checklist for an Emergency Situation
Overdue Baby
Breach Baby
Caesarean Birth
Welcoming your Baby Exercise
A Ceremony for Welcoming and Blessing your Baby
Post Natal Care for the Mother's Body
The Four Step Birth Release Action Plan
Birth Acceptance Exercise
Birth Release Meditation
Examples of Postnatal Mantras

7 Clear Parent
Exercise for Parenting Approach
Visualisation for Healthy Breastfeeding
Meditation For Being Present with your Child
Calming an Anxious Baby
Meditation to Calm Mother and Child

Part Three - The Forty Day Programme
The Ten Step Birth Manifestation Action Plan
7 Rules for the Forty Day Programme
Birth Mantras from 32 Weeks
Visualisation of Mantras
A Manifestation Meditation
Examples of Pregnancy Daily Practise
7 Key Pointers for Manifesting your Sacred Birth
7 Key Pointers for Creating Good Vibrations in The Aquarian Age

Programme Guide

Your Birthing Journal It is recommended that you read the book and follow the exercises in chronological order with a pen and notebook to hand, making notes on any feelings that arise as you go along. Follow the exercises in order unless it is clearly stated that you should leave an exercise until you reach the Forty Day programme in Part Three.

Examples taken from birth journals are written like this.

When to Start Start the book at any point but look to starting Part Three from around week 32 of your pregnancy. This is approximate. You need to allow enough time to follow the exercises properly in the lead up to commencing the Forty Day programme in Part Three. You may wish to repeat the exercises in Part One and Two many times before starting Part Three.

Your Birth Altar Set up a birth table or altar with inspirational images, stones, crystals, fresh flowers, ornaments – anything that is special to you. This is where you keep your Birth Power Mantras, drawings, special creams and oils filled with light, birthing journal and this book. If you decide to have a scan, place your image here alongside images of birthing angels that you have found or drawn, or images that represent how you want your birth to be. You can place a happy, healthy body scan drawing here. Use this special place to do your meditations and to follow the forty day programme. I recommend you have an image of your choice to represent the Goddess Mother here who will hold you through this most special time.

Daily Practice This is your daily 'ME' time to fill you up and bathe within. As an approximate guide, from the very start allow time here daily to practise self worth, with one hand on your heart and the other on your womb, and just tuning into yourself, your baby and your inner worth and self listening. Then from week 22, allow a minimum of half an hour daily practice space every day with any exercises in this book. Then from week 32, allow around a minimum of one hour a day. This is just an approximate guide. You need to arrange your lifestyle to fit this in now. This is important preparation for the birth of your baby and you owe this to your family, to your baby and to yourself. Remember this sacred quiet time is about creating relaxing 'ME' time in a sacred quiet meditative space. It is always possible to find time each day for yourself and your coming baby, and if not, it is essential that you look at why not.

Ideas for Daily Practice before your Altar

Open the space with a candle, crystals, essential oil and so on. Invoke any guides or angels whom you want to be present.

Thanks List five things that you are grateful for and / or say five "well done for" statements to your children, self or partner.

Forgiveness Release any tension by forgiving yourself and others for irritations today, forgive five things (there is a more in depth exercise in the book on forgiveness)

Grounding Simply ask for grounding, or invoke White Light or breathe in Light from the sun into your heart. Imagine white or gold Light forming a golden sphere around you, or imagine a six pointed white crystal star around you. This will tune you into the Earth's crystal grid. To ground yourself, imagine roots from your feet going deep into the Earth's crystal centre, or imagine a White Light circling in a clockwise direction up from your feet to your crown seven times then back down through your head, into the Earth.

Relax and Nourish Breathe in the good and breathe out any tension. Massage your body. Chant words of self love on the out-breath such as "I am beautiful, I am loved", or simply, "All is well".

Connection Ask for messages in dreams, and ask the universe to guide and provide, knowing that God is your source. Connect to your Higher Self, your baby and your body by talking to them with positive language. They will do as you ask them to!

Presence and Worth start practising self listening to all you feel and practising inner worth by saying any self value and self love mantras that come naturally to you with one hand on your heart and one on your womb, and just feel yourself giving value to all you feel and are.

Meditate and Tune In follow the book exercises and the birthing programme. This may involve wanting to sit and say your affirmations, rehearse your birth, reflect and draw in your journal, follow visualisations, just sit and be with yourself, your body and your baby and so on. Keep the focus on the Divine Mother using the image on the back cover.

Close the Space After giving thanks, close the circle by grounding and protecting, closing your chakras by imagining flower petals closing over each chakra. Blow out candles with a closing word (for example - Amen, Om, So it Is or Sat Nam)

Importance of Just Being Or you can spend your daily preparation in your sacred space just being, just relaxing in front of your birth table.

Remembering the River

*The river was like a mother holding and sustaining all life
lapping with her tides
whatever, and whomever unconditionally.
The ducks swam in her waters, held and nurtured.
Swans, fish, birds, frogs, plants
eating, fighting, sleeping; all held by her tides,
her arms softly lulling and sustaining and holding.
Oh, to feel this mother inside, supporting and holding us…
to feel her tides within us, holding, supporting
nourishing us in all we do.
Being held.*

*Oh! To be this essence!
To be the river within as we nurture our child,
loving unconditionally whilst
letting our waters
flow clear.*

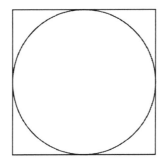

Introduction

The Mirror Concept

As within, so without
As we think, so we are
As we believe, so we will be

In the Bhagavad Gita, Lord Krishna says to Arjuna,

"Thy business is with action only, never with its fruits;
so let not the fruit of action be thy motive,
nor be thou to inaction attached.
Perform action, Dhananjaya,
dwelling in union with the divine,
renouncing attachments,
and balanced evenly in success and failure:
equilibrium is called yoga"

(Gita 11, 47-48)

and thus,
dwelling in union with the divine
is key to all
then the music flows
the cow bears milk
and yet how much milk or when and how
is not of any matter
it is the flow of music we immerse within
and this has one source only
to dwell in union with the divine
then the waters and the milks shall flow

Manifestation "Letting-go whilst acting as-if"

Everything is energy and frequency
Belief and emotion is a result of energy
This inner frequency magnetises to it
things of the same frequency
The inner core inner beliefs and emotions
thus create the reality around us

What is Manifestation?

Christa followed this programme. Her journal notes included:

"...Making an idea real. Consciously making your positive desires real and appear in form, through using the power of the mind. Looking at what you think and believe to be possible, with awareness that what is happening within you reflects what is happening outside of you – and vice versa...."

What would yours say? Jot down a few words right now, or have a quick reflection before continuing.

Manifestation and empowerment go hand in hand, since to fully live in your whole power you need to own, follow, speak and live your truth, regardless of other people's desires. This includes being aware of your subconscious conditioned inner beliefs and inner emotions, that hold a frequency within you.

In order to make your dreams manifest and to live within your full power, it is essential to be able to do what you want and follow your flow. Anything that prevents you from 'following your flow' causes dis-harmony or dis-ease, and arises from a consciousness of lack rather than from one of abundance.

We are all worthy of abundance. The problems of the world stem from people doing what they believe that they 'have to do' rather than what they actually really want to do: from people believing that they are victim to others or to circumstance, rather than realising that they have a choice and a voice.

Imagine what the world would be like if we all felt free and secure enough to to 'do our thing (respectfully), whatever we wanted as we felt was right for us, rather than pleasing others and living according to other people's insecurities. It is interesting that when we live in connection with out intuition of what our soul desires (as opposed to false desires and hungers based on lack and need) then our flow will naturally benefit and respect all others around us too (and anyone challenges will be so because they are living in lack and need).

Healthy relationships enable both partners to fully express who they are. We then come together from a place of in-power rather than looking towards each other for that power and fulfilment (codependency). The latter will simply create ego power struggles. If you fear giving another person freedom, then that relationship is based on fear and need.

We are the source of our selves. When we look to others to fill us then this is codependency and unhealthy enmeshment. Most humans have been taught to get fulfilment and energy from without, from some source out there. This might be other people or consumption of things (it is a materialistic culture that we have been programmed into). So we all have to re learn how to fill direct from source within us. For example, the Celestine Prophecy outlines some key 'drama roles' that most of us use in order to fill up, when living without awareness.

Some desires are based on false desire or need, they are ego-dominated. If the energy is not right and things are forced, you will know. It is important to follow deep intuitive soul callings rather than whims or 'false desires' stemming from inner needs to repress trauma, and you will know the difference if you are honest with yourself. Does my body really want this sugar or is that a false desire? Do I really not want to go there or is that a fear resistance? Deep within, you know.

Many people believe that desire keeps people bound to "karma" and prevents them from being whole and present with "God": if you desire something then you are unhappy with how things are right now. This is a reference to lower level false desires. And yet it is true that when we let go of the want for anything, the fruits of the dream, then we manifest them anyhow. But we need to be full in each moment first. Think of the teenage girl wanting the boy to call and he never does and when she releases the yearning, the phone rings.

The four noble truths of the Buddha state that everything is suffering (or leads to dissatisfaction) since we live in a world bound by desire. To break suffering is simply to break away from desire. This does not mean removing yourself from desire absolutely and living naked in a cave, feeding on plants. After all, it is inspiration that gets humanity out of bed in the morning. Rather, it means removing yourself from the *attachment* to a desire. You need to give up the 'need' for the outcome, to end the suffering. Letting go of the 'need' for something. It is the 'need' which is pain derived and ego driven, but desire as a form of soul creative flow is healthy when it has no 'need' for a specific outcome.

The innate human urge to create and to inspire can be confused with a need for fulfilment, or to repress hidden trauma with consumption, which is ego and pain derived as opposed to from a clear inspiration. So you understand how this is another paradox of manifestation: this 'need to have and to create' could be either an intuitive calling or it could be a form of escape from the emptiness within, a need to fill up the void. And you can understand that ironically, fulfilment will come by accepting 'what is', whilst simultaneously being open to what could be.

So being separate to 'Goddess' or the 'Light Source' causes a need for fulfilment – a need to fill up the empty space. This is done in our society by external consumption, seeking fulfilment through desires which lead to cravings and addictions to people and substances (both emotional and physical). More food, more cigarettes, more sex, more chocolate, more ideas, more things to do, a better home, a better car, a better dress, he's not good enough...looking outside to fill the (w)hole and a quick fix to make better in some way.

If you follow your true callings and follow where the energy flows (in regard to people, events and places, only go and see whatever seems to "hum" for you), then you will find yourself in the right places at the right time, and at the same time find that any ego dominated desires do not appeal to you. The first way to do this is with intuition: following the places that are light for you (they shine) and the things that make you feel good.

However, it is not always that simple because we have root pattens, traumas, blocks, survival programs and so forth locked away in the subconscious that we are not even aware of, creating the same patterns in our lives. So no matter how much we affirm our way forth and how much light filling we do, we might still end up repeating old patterns. Until we do the inner work. When we do the inner work to target the root of these survival programs or ancestral patterns, then we can shift the entire frequency from within, into something new.

So you see that there is much paradox here! The less desire you have and the more you are happy in the now, the more likely it is that abundance will come your way and your manifestation for a particular desire will take place. As well as accepting the present state of being, we also need to clear inner subconscious blocks, whilst at the same time uplifting into higher states and flowing with intuition.

The road to manifesting a desire leads to the path of non-attachment to desire (letting go of your need and attachment for the desire), since that is necessary for the desire to manifest. And yet whilst letting go of the desire, and being happy with everything as it is right now, we also work on the subconscious traumas that hold us back from realising it. I like to say to my students that the path of healing is not about making ourselves better in some way, but it is about releasing the parts of us that don't think we are perfect just as we are already.

So first you understand the importance of 'letting go' once you have put out your desire for something, and just being happy with the now. Give up the craving to be full by filling up from within rather than by attempting to fulfil a desire and the desire will manifest anyway, even though it no longer matters if it does or does not.

So the paradox of this programme is that it says, on the one hand, manifest your birth dream! Then, on the other hand, it says surrender to it and let it be as it is right now even if that is not as you desire. Give in to it. Your baby will have his or her own karma to play out in this birth too, although you can affect this with healing and shining what I call 'womb light' and releasing any blocks.

Therefore you can now understand that the key to manifestation is to
NAME your clear intention,
ALLOW any blocks to surface to be seen and healed,
LET GO of the attachment and the desire,
ACCEPTING what already is and connecting to you fulfilment within right now,
ACTING AS IF your desire is in a reality,
ALLOWING change to take place if it is for the greatest good
TRUSTING AND KNOWING it is all manifest already as Goddess intends.

The universe is a mirror, and if you act as-if, it will be-come. Throughout this book I refer to this seemingly contradictory concept as *"letting go whilst acting as if"*. *'Acting as if you already have it'* can allow the need and attachment and desire itself to dissolve. We can help ourselves to find that feeling of being absolutely fulfilled and 'wanting for nothing' by doing the inner work on targeting blocks and emotional traumas or survival beliefs, to alter the inner frequencies that we resonate. This way we magnetise new ones, but without the 'need'.

And so, if a desire is something you want because you believe it will make you feel better or happier in some way, remember that it is important that for a desire to come true, you must be happy first, and thus not *attached* to the outcome.

But you also need to BELIEVE it will come true. You WANT and you BELIEVE, and then you LET GO and ALLOW. Belief is an important part of manifesting.

Some people work hard to earn the money to enable them to do the things they want in order to be happy. Most successful people however are just happy and they do whatever they want and trust that the rest will follow. It is all about trust. Turn it around. You choose. Instead o being the victim you choose to be the empowered creator in each and every moment. Always coming out of reaction and taking things to sacred space.

If you follow your truth, you will be enabling others to be in their power too. Let's say you do not want to meet someone this afternoon although you made the arrangement weeks earlier. It does not feel right and you do not want to be there. Worried about letting them down, you contact them anyway. They might say, "It's lucky you phoned because...." Or they may be cross that they have been "let down" but actually find later that "it was so lucky that ... cancelled or ...would not have happened". Even if they don't ever realise it, it will have been for their greater good for reasons unknown. If on the other hand you ignore the feeling and go and meet them, later you will know why: " I *knew* I shouldn't have gone...."

If you follow your truth you will always be in the right place at the right time, even if on the surface it does not look right.

There is an old story called "Good Luck, Bad Luck...Who can tell?"

A father and his son owned a farm. They did not have many animals, but they did own a horse. One day the horse ran away.
"How terrible, what bad luck," said the neighbours.
"Good luck, bad luck, who knows?" replied the farmer.
Several weeks later the horse returned, bringing with him four wild mares.
"What marvellous luck," said the neighbours.
"Good luck, bad luck, who knows?" replied the farmer.
The son began to learn to ride the wild horses, but one day he was thrown and broke his leg.
"What bad luck," said the neighbours.
"Good luck, bad luck, who knows?" replied the farmer.
The next week the army came to the village to take all the young men to war. The farmer's son was still disabled with his broken leg, so he was spared. "Good luck, bad luck, who knows?"

The law of Dharma says that we have taken manifestation in physical form to fulfil a purpose and find our unique talent. Sometimes finding and following your unique calling is not easy and can be challenging. This is where you can ask spiritual helpers for guidance, whatever faith you follow.

It is challenging knowing that you are master of your own universe here to live your unique talent: that you can have anything you desire if you ask for it. No one is a victim. Everything that happens is a reflection of your thoughts and emotions. Realising this is a big part of the first step to empowerment. Many people find this concept challenging, especially when looking at war situations, but there are people who have had 'lucky' escapes and miracles, or 'made it big' from nothing.

The concept of emotions within creating your reality, is fundamental to the concept of manifestation. It is vital to start being aware of your emotions and finding the root energy behind them in order to shift them. We have to do this outside of the conscious mind and go into the sub conscious.

This is how you make your wishes come true.

These are all big concepts. Following them is a lifetime's journey. There are layers upon layers. This is a journey that is exemplified by pregnancy and imminent birth and parenting, since you want to give your children the best you can and also because you are wide open when you are pregnant to the emotions within and the ethers around you. This is wonderful because it means that you are the most open for healing when you are pregnant. So if seeming 'negative' emotions arise they are wonderful opportunities to get to the root cause for healing ancestral patterns through generations. You have the power by doing this work to affect 7 generations back and 7 generations forward! Pregnant women can accelerate their life's journey since they are so open to soak up spirit. This is why dolphins are so attracted to pregnant women. Indeed pregnant women are sometimes not allowed on dolphin trips as it is unfair on the other tourists: all the dolphins swim only to her" she is an energetic magnet.

When you are pregnant you are an energetic magnet!

Being within your full power and preparing to make manifest your birthing wishes, is not only about manifesting a beautiful birth and perhaps even a painless and joyful easy one, but it is also about healing your ancestors and creating new ways of living for the future generations! This is your birth right and your birth opportunity as a birthing mother.

Sadly our current culture has not recognised the primary importance of birthing in our power as the creation of smooth and happy birth, nor does this culture even recognise what it actually means to be 'in our power'. So it is up to us to take matters into our own hands and take full power back for our own births. And reclaim our power as women.

So this is the invitation to heal yourself in order to imagine your highest outcome for you and for your baby. You also need to be clear and light with good food and a clear body in order to enable the manifestation to take place. The more clear you are, the more magic can happen. It all begins with self love, which takes you to a place of full power which in turn enables manifestation and birth to be clear.

This book is aimed to take you through this journey of both clearing out the old and creating the clear inner connection, before you reach the manifestation programme itself in the final part.

Sacred Birth - Intuitive Birth

What is Intuitive Birth?

Christa's notes included:

"...Birthing from within, from a place of inner knowing, from our instincts, from the place where your body knows what to do more than any understanding or knowledge that the rational mind could dream up, trusting your baby knows what to do, faith in millions of years of nature, faith in "God" and knowing that your intuition will tell you everything, from what position to what herb. Doing everything we can to be in a place where we clearly just know with our gut and being respected and honoured and supported by those around to follow that..."

What would your notes say? Jot some more words in your birth journal...

What is Sacred Birth?

Christa's notes include:

"...A "beautiful" birth, whatever "beautiful" means for you, is surely sacred. Birthing your baby from a place that is turned inwards towards "God", whatever "God" means for you, or whatever religion you employ, since God is a place of beauty. Trusting your inner guidance and employing gentle methods of relaxation within a quiet and respectful environment. Faith and surrender in your body, baby and inner guidance; aware that your instincts are the primary governing factor towards healthy birth and relaxation. Avoiding invasive intervention and stress / tension where possible since this creates pain and trauma for both mother and baby..."

What about yours...?

Why choose Intuitive Techniques for Sacred Birth?

Sacred birthing is about hearing your intuition. Intuition (or the voice of "God") will guide you to open your light womb up wide in the way that you want and need to do. Your mind cannot know how to do this, it is intuitive, it comes from deep within you.

When you are cut off from your intuition, **fear blocks the birth hormones** from being released and prevents you from opening up, which leads to pain and intervention whilst you lend your power to someone who tells you what you need to do.

If you follow your intuition, you do not need to be afraid as you will know all that you need to do when you need to do it. Ironically, the very thing you are afraid of – a painful or 'bad' birth, is the very thing that causes it: whilst fear blocks the birth hormones, relaxation enables the great opening to occur.

So this Manifest Sacred Birth Programme is mainly based on Intuitive Birthing Techniques because intuition is the voice of the Higher Self. For example, if you are still and in tune, your hand will intuitively reach to catch a falling glass long before your mind has realised it will fall. If your mind is still and your emotions in check, then you can sink to a deeper place beyond ego, desire, thought chatter, other people's desires, your own false desires, shoulds, 'what ifs', fears and so forth, directly into a place of stillness and all-knowing. This is where you can birth in tune with your body's signals; your body knows what to do, it knows how to grow a baby and how to birth a baby; it is your mind which does not.

I **have coined the term 'Intuitive Birth' since it suggests that there is no right or wrong way to birth**, but focuses on birthing in the way that is right for the unique individual. Since we are all individuals with unique faces, bodies, habitats, relationships, homes, children, lifestyle situations, desires and needs, past experiences, past lives, future lives and so on, only our intuition can know what is in our own best interests. For this reason, we can never say "you need to do this or that" to another. All we can do is learn the tools to be with our own instincts. A doctor cannot know our bodies as well as our instinct can. Therefore we can never judge another on how they birthed and we can never pressure ourselves to do it well or the 'right' way.

So, since we are all unique, Intuitive Birth does not advocate birthing at home but focuses on birthing from your intuition, wherever that may lead you. This book does focus on home birth since I believe that it is easier to access your intuition from a quiet, sacred, safe, warm environment. If your intuition says "Go to hospital!" and you are sure that this is not fear (as explored in the book), then you can learn later on how to create a sacred space even in a hospital waiting room.

There are so many accepted myths around birth that we buy into without realising or thinking about it. One in particular is that birth is painful.

Birth does not need to be painful!

If you are relaxed, your birth can be easy, and your body will be so full of endorphins that you can actually enjoy the sensation of opening to the right shape for your body and your baby. This has been proven, and you can watch clips of so-called 'ecstatic births' on the internet (see Birth Into Being, Elena Tonetti, in Appendix). There are many natural childbirth organisations springing up at the moment that are based on this realisation and many methods of accessing this relaxation are becoming available - hypnosis birth, massage birth, active birth. This book brings most of these ways together into one unique programme with a focus on the sacred - mantra, meditation, visualisation and ceremony.

Birth is a powerful rite of passage for men as well as for women; it is a time for men to become empowered and to grow. As a man you are a vital part of the birthing process, and it is essential that like a woman you learn to reconnect to your divine Higher Self and be a part of the birthing process fully within your power too, whatever that role means for you.

And let's not forget that birthing is the first step in parenting. Intuitive birth is the first step in creating and nourishing an emotionally happier and thus highly advanced child. Each step affects another. Intuitive Parenting is therefore discussed towards the end of the book and there are examples of evidence of the beneficial long term effects of Sacred Birth in the appendix. Our children are our future. Our future relies on the next generation taking us forward into new ways of living, doing, being, communicating and thinking which in turn will have a global impact on our environment and planet. It is up to parents today to teach our children these new ways of being. Parents are the key to evolution for our planet, and as parents-to-be you are about to do the most important job in the world. By parenting in sacred ways you are giving your child and your world the best gift you can.

The techniques in Manifest Sacred Birth are tried and tested by myself. This book is an amalgamation of my own birthing journals. I wrote down the meditations and affirmations that arose in my pregnancies and births and it just turned into a book, written mostly whilst being constantly interrupted by babies or in snatches of time whilst they slept. Even though it was challenging to find the time to write the methods down, it seemed like sacrilege if I did not share them with others. So it is my wish to present tools for the empowerment of both women and men in their birthing space, to prevent a feeling of pain and trauma but instead encourage joy and strength. I hope to help you reconnect with your intuition so that you can birth from your full power. I feel passionate about giving alternative ways of birthing to the accepted but barbaric, invasive, disempowering, disconnected, ego-dominated, painful, fear-inducing, belittling and unnecessary birthing methods that are currently in practise in our so called 'civilised' culture.

When I was first pregnant, I knew little of these birthing concepts, and during my pregnancy I went from expecting a hospital birth to asking for a magical empowering home birth. Along the way, it became apparent that I was learning much more than how to give birth in the way I wanted. I was healing myself, relationships, ancestors, and much more. For the first time I started to live in my truth more fully than ever. Being pregnant and having children also meant that I had an *excuse* to do what I wanted, say "no" to people, and to actually live my truth!

In my first pregnancy, I thought I was going to birth at the local small midwifery centre and was preparing for that. As the pregnancy progressed, however, the more yoga, visualisation and meditation I did, the stranger it felt to do that. When I became three weeks 'overdue', I came under a great deal of pressure from medical staff and was classed as high risk. At that stage, I had no choice but to say "I will birth at home then." They panicked but it was my legal right. I had attended routine scans and tests (something I wouldn't do now) and had been told that my baby was high risk for Down's Syndrome: 1 in 200 chances. Later, I had a scan for something else and was told I was low risk: again 1 in 200 chances. So I knew that sometimes the panic from the medical professionals did not have any foundation in logic and it felt rigid and fearful, where as the decision to birth at home felt right, clear and empowered.

As time was passing, I was told it was a danger and that the placenta was starting to decay but I knew it was okay and it was not right for me to have intervention. I had a lot of pressure for intervention and I was moving further away from medical supervision due to some strange instinct. At one point I did compromise and go for a check up and a nurse examined me and tried to break my waters, but after I had made time in a private moment in the toilet for a meditation and prayer, the nurse then couldn't find my cervix. She was embarrassed by this absurdity and sent me home to return the next day. That same afternoon I was examined by my gentle midwife at home who found my cervix but did not try and break my waters. By then I was strong enough to be clear that I did not want that.

Then, when I finally accepted my fear of a hospital intervention, and the fight to maintain my space, I went into the final stages of birth at home. Then the idea of leaving the birth dance in candlelight to get into a car and go somewhere else seemed absurd, and luckily I was empowered enough to trust and follow my instinct and stay at home with my partner's gentle support. A midwife arrived but did not believe that I was about to birth as it was 'too early on'. In fact, it turned out that I had actually been in birth for days without anyone realising, as it was so gentle because of all my meditations! I birthed my baby girl myself and caught her myself as she glided out complete in her waters (exactly like my mantras, due to concerns about a herpes infection I had previously had) whilst the midwife was in the other room doing paper work. All was well. Later, the Midwife examined me and my placenta and saw a major artery which would have been have ruptured had the waters been broken, which they attempted to do only a few days before. My excuse to goto the toilet and do prayer in there worked for me. That would have been life threatening for us both. They said it was a miracle I hadn't got my waters broken so that we were both okay.

By my next unexpected pregnancy the following year, I was empowered enough to know that I wanted a sacred home birth and how to create this. However I had new issues that arose around the birth - such as worries about my daughter and relationship issue with my husband. Using the mediations from which I developed the programme in this book, I managed to heal these issues both before, and also during the actual birth process itself, and continued to have an unassisted, beautiful, sacred home birth. The midwife was in the other room, my husband had been wonderful at protecting my space after he noticed my voice become self conscious when she came to 'observe' me and things slowed down. He requested that she leave the room and things progressed again when I was left alone and able to focus on visual meditations alone to work through issues and get into a trance again. He had sent her colleague home telling her she was not required. We were lucky to have a local midwife that understood our approach, and if we hadn't we probably would have just gone it alone completely, rather than have someone in the room imposing their beliefs and presence into the space. For me, that seemed like having sex while someone in a white coat stood watching and taking notes on your behaviour. How do you orgasm like that? After all, birth is like an enjoyable orgasm if you are birthing without tension.

Two days after my second birth, when we were in vulnerable and sleepless states, we 'accidentally' allowed a doctor in to examine our baby and ended up in hospital having our baby examined due to the doctor's fear of how we had birthed. Our baby was fine and I knew he was fine, he was waking up to the world slowly and taking his time, so he had not yet urinated. But the doctor managed to install fear into me when I was very open and vulnerable so despite all my inner work, we headed there to have him checked. The visit to hospital did disrupt our post baby bubble but it was an interesting lesson. He was fine and urinated as soon as we arrived so luckily we went home fast. The midwife came to visit a few days later, and was confused about the situation saying that in the circumstance we had been in, doctors usually leave longer before sending a baby to hospital. I later discovered that the doctor who visited us was also a politician who had was vehemently anti home birth. She was outraged at our set up and it challenged her. But we could not blame, we were the ones who listened and taken on this fear and gone to hospital when deep down we KNEW that our baby was fine.

It is very easy to get caught up in other people's fears, needs and expectations, especially when it comes to the health and safety of our children. This is deep emotional territory that people have strong feelings about. The only tool we have to help us know what we need to do is our instinct. Likewise it can be very difficult to distinguish between fear and instinct when surrounded by the medical profession - do I really need to go to hospital? Sometimes we do and our instinct, not our fear, senses this. For this reason, I have included the meditations in this book to help you to distinguish between instinct and fear.

Birthing sacredly is about setting up protection with visualisation, it is about affirming mantras to protect and create a happy situation, it is about ways of being able to tune in so that we can decipher for ourselves whether we need or want an intervention - and about making choices because we know they are right, rather than from fear of health and safety risk assessments that may not have a scientific basis at all.

It is about being in a clear enough space to decipher between fear based false desires (from a place of what-if worries, focusing on negative outcome when there need not be any, hurt, pain, ego, need, desire) and intuitive light-connected healthy desires (from a place of clarity, inner knowing, Light, positivity, instinct).

I hope that this book enables you to find your power and make manifest your dream birth, enabling you and your family to live fully in abundance and light. May we create a world of great wise souls making way for a Golden Age, living in harmony with each other and the planet.

The mother holds the power for the future.

Finally, it must be highlighted that the purpose of this book is always *intuitive* birth. Please do not heed any advice that does not feel right. Always ask yourself before taking anything on board: "Is this my truth? Is this right for me?" Likewise, before making any decision say to yourself: "If I loved myself (and my baby) I would …" and "Will this action lead me / us towards sacredness?" The tools in this book will help you to access your subconscious to tell you the answers you need.

For manifestation to occur, and for our births to be beautiful, we need to be clear in our bodies and our energy. We need to be full of **womb-light**. Manifest Sacred Birth is therefore in three parts: firstly you will learn how affirmations work, then you will clear away any emotional energetic inner blocks with intuitive birthing techniques, then finally you will be ready to manifest.

My Love to you,
Ishtara xx

Book Note: This book is at times purposefully repetitive to transmit fundamental positive birthing messages firmly into the subconscious mind.

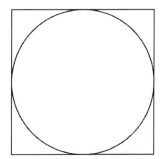

Part One

Your Birth Power Mantras

Mantra and Japa

Mantras are based on the concept that you are what you think and feel and believe, so the world reflects your thoughts, feeling and beliefs. Your thoughts, feelings and core subconscious beliefs become your truth and will attract your experiences in the world. There are no accidents, only reflections of energy. Mantras create energetic ripples to pave open the way forth. In these ten steps you will learn how to tune into your deep internal beliefs and subconscious inner most emotions and transform them into positive ones in order to make space for your sacred birth. This way we work from the subconscious and the inner quantum field, and not just using general affirmations from the 'outer'. This is much more powerful. It addresses and targets the inner energy directly to shift the outer world.

Mantra is a sound, syllable, word or group of words that is considered capable of "creating transformation" (spiritual transformation). Mantras that are in a different language (Hindu, Sikh) can be thousands of years old using sounds that are specific seed sounds scientifically designed to make specific changes in the body. In some forms of yoga like Kundalini Yoga, one can follow a kriya (set of postures) with a mantra at the same time for specific aims such as being relaxed, creating abundance, removing obstacles and so on.

When one chants a specific set of words that positively resonate internally, in any language, with a specific reason in mind, this can be called Mantra. Mantras spoken in one's mother tongue (as opposed to Sikh or Hindu) are also known as 'affirmations' or 'positive truth statements'. If one chants a mantra in the mother tongue it is important to find the correct words given to you form your subconscious or the ones that really resonate for you, so that the change can take place, rather than just saying aloud a positive affirmation that may not resonate and does not directly addressing the inner emotional cause. You need to FEEL them as you say them. You can even give them colour or a symbol. It is important to create your own mantras rather than just picking them out of a book, unless they intuitively resonate and stand out for you when you look through a list (such as examples ones presented in this book). It is essential to feel and breathe the mantra, rather than just say it, and tune into its positive quality rather than focusing too much on the pain one may experience and be releasing.

The next steps focus on creating your own unique mantras from your own unique subconscious for your own unique birth, as you imagine it to be, and there are also a few key ancient mantras listed in Step Ten.

Japa is a concept of the Vedic sages that incorporates mantras as one of the main forms of worship (Puja), whose ultimate end is seen as liberation (Moksha). Essentially, Mantra Japa means repetition of mantra, and it has become a practice of most Hindu variations, from the various schools of Yoga to Tantra. Japa involves repetition of a mantra over and over again, usually in cycles of auspicious numbers (in multiples of three), the most popular being 108. For this reason, Hindu malas (bead necklaces) contain 108 beads and a head bead (sometimes referred to as the guru bead). The devotee performing japa counts each bead using his/her fingers as he/she repeats the chosen mantra. Having reached 108 repetitions, if he/she wishes to continue with another cycle of mantras, the devotee must turn the mala around, without crossing the head bead, and repeat. You can use japa (recitation of mantra) as you go about your every day life, either by your own spoon tongue or chanting along with you own recording or musical recordings of your choice, bringing your cared practise into the every day.

Guide to the Ten Steps

These ten steps are designed to create your own personal birthing mantras.

Follow the Ten Steps slowly in chronological order.

Once you have completed them properly, you may continue with the rest of the book.

You will return to repeat them in Part Three as part of the Birth Manifestation Programme.

The Ten Step Magical Birthing Mantra Creation is based on this understanding and three key statements:

Mantra Creation is about intention: connect to your intention, that which you 'want to create' within yourself first, then clear out the blocks, and give it to God, knowing it will be reflected back by events and others around you

1. You CAN have anything you want.

2. You just need to fully BELIEVE it.

3. And that you are WORTHY of it in order for it to happen.

Step One

Thoughts and Feelings Right Now

The next 10 steps will help you to create your own unique mantras from your own unique subconscious for your own unique birth, as you imagine it to be, and there are also a few key ancient mantras listed in Step Ten. These mantras will also become part of your birth intention.

Before you start to create them by following the 10 steps, first write down a birth intention from your heart or womb, in a few simple sentences. You can then use the 10 steps to turn this birth intention from a blind hope, into words that hold great power and magic.

So write your intention as it is right now, and put it before your altar. As you feel into your birth intention, the first stage is to start to both gently become aware of all your thoughts, feelings and beliefs about all parts of your life as they are right now and also asking for any blocks in your way to come forth now to bring to light for healing and resolution. You are working through the space of the inner realms, as opposed to being in the mind.

The Right Now Chart

With your intention set and put to one side, you are now to commence by tuning in and placing one hand on your heart and the other on your womb, and then when you write, do not write from the mind but from a place deep within, try to bypass your mind completely.

Note down all your first thoughts and feelings about pregnancy and birth and then continue into other aspects of your life, since everything is linked. First list everything that you think, then list everything that you feel, right now, about each area of your life. Not as you wish it to be, but as it really is right now.

This is not an exercise about what you *should* think, or what is right. It is absolutely essential that you jot down what you genuinely think and feel right now, good and bad (or better, without judgement at all), so that you can be absolutely aware of where you are right now and it is very important you write the first things that come, writing from the heart and the inner, and not from the mind, with absolutely frank honesty.

Then continue to note your thoughts and feelings both positive and negative, during the coming weeks. When anything arises, make note of it mentally and then when you have time jot it down in your birthing journal.

Stop and fill in this chart now and add any more subjects that you think may be relevant -

Right Now

Area	Feelings	Thoughts
Birth		
Pregnancy		
Children and babies		
Parenthood		
Relationships		
My partner		
My children		
My family		
My parents		
My friends		
My body		
My health		
My home		
My career		
Money and success		

Step Two

Going Beyond with Meditation

A Course in Miracles states "You have no neutral thoughts... everything you see is a result of your thoughts. There is no exception to this fact. Thoughts are not big or little, powerful or weak. They are merely true or false. Those that are true create their own likeness. Those that are false make theirs... every thought you have contributes to truth or illusion; either it extends the truth or multiplies the illusion."

Practising mindfulness or thought awareness is essential for manifestation. Try to become more aware of your thoughts, beliefs and emotions in each moment without judgement or analysis for the mind. Just gentle awareness.

Practising self-presence is essential for birth. To birth well it is necessary to retain the trance state of self presence, so start practising this now. Beyond "thinking" is "not thinking", which means just being present – being here now, and allowing all that is, with no judgement, but with self worth and value for all you feel as a human being, as child of the Goddess. This is the place you want to birth from. Being present here and now with no thought and no judgement is being one with God. This is also the place you need to be pregnant in: the present, without thoughts of the future or the birth itself – even whilst preparing for birth as practice for being present with yourself in the birth.

If you don't feel drawn to 'sit and meditate', that is fine. Instead try just to sit with yourself for a little time by the altar and feel yourself with your self worth, and that is enough. Spend the day times by coming into awareness of your thoughts and feelings as and when you can, with no judgement. You might even start to label them in a helpful loving way, such as *"having a 'what-if' thought again right now......another 'what-if' fear-based thought again, I feel this in my tummy,.....ah, a 'to-do' thought...my heart feel tight, I remember this feeling when I was 6 and...."*

Below is a meditation you can start to do in your daily birth preparation space. After practising this meditation, you can try to bring presence into everyday life. Washing up, at the traffic lights, in the post office queue, in the supermarket... whatever you are doing, try and be present with it. Whilst out walking with your partner, you may suddenly catch yourself chatting on and on about something. As soon as you become aware of this you can come back to 'here and now' and let all the thoughts go, without judgement.

None of the thoughts that arise are important - you are always only one thought away from God at any time. The more you practise presence, stillness, sitting with self listening, and being here right now without any thought, the more you will able to be present within your birth. This will help create calm and relaxation, which in turn prevents trauma and pain and enables easy birth. Saying a mantra such as *"I choose to experience this moment right now"* can help bring you instantly into the present.

"Repeating the name of God once, when mind is controlled, is equivalent to a million repetitions when the mind strays from God. You may repeat the name of God for the whole day, but if the mind be elsewhere that does not produce much result. The repetition of the name must accompany concentration." The Holy Mother, Sri Saradamani Devi

In the Bhagavad Gita, Krishna says to Arjuna "Still your mind in me, still your intellect in me, and without doubt you will be united with me forever. If you cannot still your mind in me, learn to do so through the regular use of meditation. If you lack the will for such self-discipline, engage yourself in my work, for selfless service can lead you at last to complete fulfilment. If you are unable to do even this, surrender yourself to me, disciplining yourself and renouncing the results of all your actions" (12:8/9/10/11)

This is good advice for one who finds meditation difficult: surrendering yourself to your baby and to "God" in both pregnancy and birth, by loving and worshipping yourself and your body, is selfless service and you will be guided to a beautiful birth.

It is said that just 1 minute of focused meditation is worth 20 minutes of meditation with the mind wondering around, and that 20 minutes of meditation is equivalent to several hours sleep.

Meditation for Thought Awareness and Presence

Set aside around just 20 minutes or so to sit in your daily birth preparation space or before your altar.

- Sit still and notice your breathing. Don't try to change your breathing, although it may change with your awareness. Make no judgement about your breathing (how it should be, where it should come from etc.), just sit and be as you are with full and loving acceptance of all that you are right now.

- Find a simple mantra or word to repeat with your breathing, such as " I Am Love", "Love", "God", "Relax", "my baby and me in light together" "self love self worth self belief" or any affirmation that empowers you. Just be with your mantra. Start to feel the light of the mantra enter your body in varied places and fill you.

- You may start to notice things in the room and you may start to think about them or you may feel something and start to think about that. Notice your thoughts but do not get lost and involved in them. Just be aware of each thought. Then move back into the realm of "no thought" or "presence" with your mantra. If you find it hard to let it go of a thought, then ask the universe that if this is really important that it will come to you again later, or write it down. Then release and come back to 'no thought' and 'just being'. If you get caught up in a thought for several minutes or much longer, don't worry. Just as soon as you realise, come back. Do not judge yourself as wrong, and likewise, never judge your thoughts themselves.

- You might find visualisation helpful: imagine stillness and light flowing in with your in-breath for the heavens through your crown, and when you breathe out all your thoughts and tensions release and drain out for transformation to light again. This is your go-to visualisation and practise this often through the day and bring it into the birth space.

- After a set time, return, give thanks and send loving energy to yourself and your baby.

Step Three

Birth Visualisation Exercise

Now let's think about your pregnancy and forthcoming birth in relation to your intention.

Read the three key statements again:

- You can have anything you want.
- You need to fully believe it,
- You must believe that you are worthy of it.

For the next week, carry the 3 statements around with you and keep reflecting on them.

These are big statements, so look at them closely. Read them several times and make a note of all the thoughts and feelings that arise in you.

For the next few exercises, we are going to focus on the first statement:

You can have anything you want.

Think about this in relation to your pregnancy and birth intention and the invite is to re visit it again with this in mind.

Repeat this to yourself and note down feelings. Then answer the following questions:

Do you know what you really want?
Do you *really* want it? Do you need it?
Does it light you up and make your heart sing?
If there were no obstacles and you could have anything you wanted in a perfect world, what would the birth be like?
Is it for the highest good? Is it a loving desire or an ego desire?
What does this make you feel?
Do you believe this is possible or not?
How does this statement reflect on your past?
What about your future?
Do you think it is selfish to have all your needs met?
Do you think it is okay?
Do you think it is possible?

Take your time and just sit with the statement, feeling it and reflecting on how it makes you feel.

Now focus on what you want in your birth: What do YOU *really* want in your birth space?

To help you think about this, write two columns in your birthing journal and call them "within" and "without".

Start both columns with the words "I love myself therefore…." before describing at length how your birth feels within and how it will be without.

WITHIN This means the feeling and the vibes of your birth. Write down key words that are important to you and really feel the vibe of the birth. You might note at this point what you want as well as what you fear or feel might happen. These are two different things and it is important to be clear in the difference.

WITHOUT Now think about the birth environment: what it will be like in the outer world? For example, where and who with? Once again be clear about what you really want and what you believe might happen. Again write key words.

Now amalgamate the columns as you write down everything you can think of for your dream birth both within and without. Let your pen write and write and get everything down. This can also be called automatic writing as you let your heart write for you without thinking too much. You can edit later. There is an example birth plan with both Within and Without to refer to later in the Birth Chapter in Part Two, but for now, just go with your instincts.

Take the time to really feel what you want inside of you, as opposed to what you *think* you should want, what you believe should happen or what is realistically possible. Forget any preconceptions of what birth looks like or feels like, and forget what is possible or not in terms of your current life situation. That is not relevant here. This is about dreaming and thinking as if anything is possible. Make believe for a while. Have fun.

Maybe you realise that actually you really want to birth on a Hawaiian beach in front of the sunset, or in a water pool with your lover, outside, surrounded by incense and flowers. In the sea with dolphins, at home with your children, alone in your bedroom, in a tepee by a river and a fire, being massaged by your mother, chanting with your lover, in a birthing centre that is near to your home, in a retreat centre far away from your home and from other people, laughing with joy, silent with sacred honour, making yourself orgasm with enjoyment, moving around on all fours, dancing to your favourite music alone, high in the mountains on a full moon….

Don't be afraid to reach for the stars. See the fears but go beyond them into what you really yearn for in your birth.

For example, did it occur to you that it is possible to birth without pain?

Take your time here. This is the key starting point for creating your beautiful birth.

Some questions to ask yourself might include:

- Where do you want to birth?
- Who with?
- What will it feel like?
- Will there be any people present? Who?
- What "vibes" will be around?
- What will the space look like?

- How long will it take?
- Will you be hot or cold? What will you be wearing?
- Will you move or be still?
- What position do you like?
- Will you have snacks present? What?
- Will you birth in day or at night?
- What sort of sounds will there be?
- Will you make sound?
- How will you announce your birth to others and what will the message look like?

….and most importantly, what does it feel like???

Remember, this is about dreaming, not about what you believe is or is not possible, nor how it is in your current real life situation.

Once again, take the next week to reflect on this whilst continuing with the next steps. This is an exercise that will be constantly developing for you.

I suggest writing at least 2 x A4 pages of how you want your pregnancy and birth to be.

Being as exact and defined as possible.

Do not follow step 4 on the same day as step 3. It is essential to first think about and feel what you want. Once you have thought about it, continue to step 4, also continuing your meditation exercises.

Step Four

'Tuning In' rather than 'Imposing Upon'

Now that you know what you really and truly want, we will now look at the difference between imposing ideas onto your pregnancy, birth, baby and children instead of flowing with the right energy from within… whilst also allowing your dream to manifest in its own beautiful flow.

We must allow a flower to open her petals in the way it wants to, at its ripe and perfect time, rather than forcing them to open in the ways and at the time that we think they should be.

An example of mind-imposing in birth might be Jessica's fixation with birthing in water. She was absolutely determined and convinced that this was what her birth was going to be like. Inside however, she kept getting a vague hunch that it was not going to be like that. She just could not get the water sensation within and it seemed that her baby did not particularly want water either. She ignored this and kept affirming the words "my baby is born in water" as the opposing affirmation to her "negative" feelings of the baby not gliding out well. However, she really needed to listen to the feeling behind her desire for water. If she had, she would have realised that she was determined to birth this way because she was afraid that her baby would not glide out easily if she was not in the water. She missed the opportunity to work on – and perhaps heal – the deeper reasons for her hunch that water was not right for her. Also, her baby was not happy in water for reasons beyond her understanding. We do not always have access to all the information, but we do have access to our intuition, which is always right and not to be confused with fear, as examined later on in this book. Jessica could have affirmed "my baby glides out smoothly and easily in the way that is right for all of us". In the end she did not have a water birth but did have a wonderful home birth. Every time she was in the water, her surges slowed right down. She was able to tune into her intuition at this point and she stopped trying to be in water! Later on, she also discovered high chemical levels in the local water systems.

Sometimes what we want is not clear and seems to conflict and become confused with our fears. The tuning in meditation below is aimed at helping with this.

Beware of imposing what you *think* it *should* be like. Keep following the flow and tuning in to your heart, rather than your mind. Ask yourself what the feeling is behind what you desire, and when you affirm, affirm the entire feeling and energy not just the thought or words.

The mantras need to come from within you. Your goal setting desires must come from within your heart and not from your mind or a false desire based in trauma.

Tuning-In Meditation

The focus for this tuning-in meditation is to now drop even deeper into your dream birth. You have now written your intention and worked out what you really want in you perfect birth, and also realised that there is an element of surrender to the flow so you are not imposing upon, but allowing it to happen, so that you are therefore tuning into your heart, body and baby to listen to what they want in the birthing space, and bypassing your mind completely.

Now we are going further.

Focus on the light of your beautiful birth and how it could be amazing for you all. In the process you may note and pick up on other issues and thoughts or resistances that pop up, possibly even seemingly completely unrelated. Do not brush these aside. Note them and then move on, returning to focus on the beautiful dream birth.

The tuning in meditation can be repeated regularly with a different focus. We could use it for any manifestation desires, issues or problems we need answers for, from health issues, conception difficulties or birth trauma to communing with our child's higher self long after they have been born!

Create some special meditation time and take the necessary steps so that you know will not be interrupted.

◦   *Sit in your beautiful space in front of a candle and crystal with some music. Take some deep breaths and let out any tension. Imagine white light holding you. Have your birth intention to hand.*

◦   *Take your time to relax. Notice your thoughts but try not to get involved with them. See the furniture or plants in the room standing still. Life goes on all around them but they keep on being still and quiet.*

◦   *When you feel relaxed, place your hand onto your heart. Imagine that your heart is breathing and breathe with it. Try not to think but instead feel all the emotions that are there. Note what they are but do not get lost in them, just try to be with them. You may feel it helps to jot down a few key words to reflect on later. If you do so, do not get lost in analysis - just a few key words is sufficient at this stage.*

◦   *Sit and breathe into your heart where your I AM Higher Self Divinity lies. Then when you feel ready, you can speak with your heart. You could say "Hello heart! Thank you for being here for me! It is nice to connect with you and be with you. Now is a time for you to let me know anything you might want me to know. I am here to focus on the birth that we are going to manifest and experience together. Have you any needs or dreams for how we could do this together?" You may also address your I AM self, your higher divinity, with a request: "Please guide me and let me be in tune with you for the coming birth".*

◦   *Try and imagine what your heart and/or I AM inner Higher Self Divinity might say. You may see pictures or images or words or imagine a voice talking or get a strong sense of knowing. You may imagine a wise being and even see what they look like, talking to you. If your heart looked like a person, what would it look like and how would it speak? Imagine it talking to you. Likewise is your Higher Self just a feeling or can you see a light or a person?*

◦   *Ask for key words for the birth to come, about both the essence and form, or names of people or Goddesses and Gods. WRITE THEM DOWN.*

○   *If you do not get anything, do not worry. That is fine. Just get a sense of your heart and your inner yearnings, hopes and dreams and Higher Self presence. Do not force them. Just sit and be in silence, just feeling.*

○   *Now you have tuned into your heart desires, you can try stating some of your dreams for your birth from stage 3 (both within and without) to your heart from your birth intention, and note what feelings arise. Sit with the feelings and if they hurt, shine light onto them. Do they correspond with your heart desires?*

○   *When you feel ready, give thanks to your heart and Higher Self and ask for any messages for your birth to keep coming to you in dreams and feelings, as well as through other people or events.*

○   *Now take some time to tune into your baby.*

○   *Place your hand over your womb and feel and imagine your beautiful baby full of light and glowing with health. Whenever you think of your baby see him/her bathed in glorious white light: a picture of health. If you are worried in any way, you may want to repeat "light, light, light" or words to that effect that work for you.*

○   *Now try and just be with your baby rather than imposing anything onto him or her. Just sit and be present with him / her for quite some time.*

○   *When you feel ready, you can talk to your baby in ways personal to you. Remember the focus of this meditation and do not get side tracked. Note anything else that crops up then return to the focus of this meditation and clearly ask your baby to respond: "I am here to see if you have any desires for this birth". After you have done this, ask your baby for any messages to come through regarding the birth and how they want it to be. Note down any thoughts or feelings about how your baby would like to birth, as well as all the other things that may have arisen.*

○   *Finally take some time to tune into your body and see what it desires for the birth.*

○   *Once again, sit and be with your body and just feel what is happening. Then when you feel ready, start talking to your body and ask it how it feels and what is happening for it right now. Return to the focus of this meditation to find out about how it would like to birth.*

○   *You can trust your baby and body to know what they are doing in the birth whether you felt like you connected to them or not. Thank and congratulate them for doing so well and affirm that you will release and hand   the birth over to them because they know what to do.*

○   *Slowly count to 3 and become aware of the room around you. Rub your hands and imagine roots into the earth to ground yourself.*

○   *Give thanks and make notes. Jot down important words and feelings and then do some automatic writing. This means just writing everything down and letting it pour out without judgement or thought. Write from your heart. You could also do some quick sketches based on the meditation. Do a quick body scan drawing as explained below. This may be a stick man with quick images and drawings of sensations around the body, or notes on how your body will feel in the birth. If you are using this tuning in meditation for health issues, you might use the body scan drawing to note down where it is light and where there are shadows or aches.*

◦ *From now onwards, be aware of events, people, images, cards, pictures, dreams, feelings… anything that rings any bells for you. You could even collect beautiful birth images for your journal. A passing comment from a stranger may set the ball rolling for the very thing that you needed. Maybe that stranger was guided to make that comment by your birthing angel. Listen and watch for signs. You can also ask for relevant dreams to come and remember to write them down in the morning.*

◦ *You are now deeply in touch with your Higher Self, your heart, body and baby for the highest good of all concerned! So be it and so it is!*

Body Scan Drawing

Close your eyes and take a few minutes to just be silent and with yourself. Take a pen and paper and draw a very quick sketch of your body with words, colours, lines, dots, dashes, symbols - just do it quickly and see what comes. You can even do this in your mind's eye without a pen and paper at all. Then you may like to correct your drawing, for example, remove things and add things until you feel that it is balanced all over. This is a form of psychic healing. You can do this for your baby too.

Automatic Writing

This is another way of tuning in.
Close your eyes and silence your thoughts. Connect to within, take deep breaths, and be clear about your focus for this exercise. Then ask your heart, intuition, angelic guides, baby or a particular bodily organ to speak. Connect to this place. Then take a pen to paper and just write freely. Don't analyse or judge your writing, just write as much as you can for as long as you can. Let anything that is seemingly irrelevant be written. It does not matter if your mind is controlling it, just write through it. If you get stuck just start with anything, even a shopping list! Just keep on going for 7 minutes or more. When you have finished, give thanks and let go. Don't analyse the words. Let them go. What is important will have either been released or will come up for you as you will subconsciously note it. Just don't analyse. This is a great way to clear the mind, tune in, release and connect. You can throw the paper away or keep it afterwards. Do whatever feels right.

Drawing your Dream Birth and Birthing Spiral

Get some blank paper and a box of coloured pens, paints, inks etc.
Now imagine your birth how you want it to be and draw it. Really tune into what you want and draw the feeling of this beautiful birth.

This can be drawn in any way, there is no wrong way. The way you do it is right for you. You could do a representative abstract image of the colours around you, or use stick people or wavy lines or a detailed image of what is in the room. You could write key words like "Trust", "Peace", "Letting Go" or names of Gods and Goddesses that you would like to be present. Or the picture may just be one line on a page… whatever feels right. Some people draw one picture and know exactly that this is it. Others find that they need to keep on drawing picture after picture until they make one that feels right.

This is your birth picture, this is what your birth will look like, hang it up in a special place and look at it daily.

Now you have drawn your dream birth, try drawing a birth spiral in colours that make you feel protected, soft, safe and like opening. This is a spiral that you can use to soothe you if you experience anxiety or pain, and to follow whilst dancing the birthing movement in your mind's eye to ensure a smooth flow for you and your baby. You might also like to draw other things to help you focus on the birth flow: a rose opening, water flowing…

Step Five

You can have anything you want

Congratulations. Now you have got to a place where you realise what you truly want in your beautiful dream birth. You have fully realised your Birth Intention which is the aim of steps 1-5.

So in this final step of this part, now it is time to summarise all this information from the previous steps and write an account of your beautiful birth in the positive tense (remove any 'won't's, 'not's or 'should's and instead say the opposing opposite positive) both WITHIN and WITHOUT.

When you have done this, look at your beautiful birth intention and say to yourself:

"This is possible. I can make this true for us right now."

This exercise is not about HOW, nor whether it is a possibility in your life right now.

Forget any hindrances, limitations or even anything that is working or helping. Instead, imagine that your dream birth is a reality right now.

Then say "I can have anything I want. I can have this. RIGHT NOW THIS IS TRUE FOR ME if I want it to be".

This is now your birth plan and the basis for your birth manifestation.

Now imagine that right now this is true for you.

As you keep on doing this, it may become apparent where your present life situation is in relation to your dream birth. You will start to think about the changes you need to make as well as notice the emotions, fears or illnesses that arise as you realise what your dream birth ideals are. The next steps are about how to deal with these fears and problems that could prevent you from manifesting your dream birth.

Step Six

Clearing Out the Blocks

We are now going to go further and help you to fully realise your birth intention.

First we need to ask for any blocks or shadows preventing this intention from being realised to rise to be seen and healed. This involves limiting throughs of your own or another's, watching your language, limiting beliefs, limiting emotions based on old survival programs, inherited patterns, or old deep seated trauma around certain themes.

Your thoughts are based on your beliefs and these are connected directly to your emotions. So we have to align your emotions, thoughts, beliefs to your birth intention so that they match energetically as the same frequency. We must do the inner work to do this.

A quick word here on trauma. When trauma happens there is a sort of soul fragmentation where a part of the soul or psyche stays in that place, that moment in time. So it is stuck on repeat in that emotion of the past, attracting things of the same frequency or vibration. Buried in the subconscious, so it is not conscious, it is happening quietly in the background. Somewhere.

So we need to find the trauma and release it to change the frequency. This is the same for anything, whether we want to heal dis - ease, or lack, or abuse patterns, or if we want to attract more of something, more abundance more joy more space. The irony with that of course is acceptance at the same time. To be fully present with what is and find the joy space abundance in the present (with presence) without needing anything out there to fill and bring it. For the source is within right now.

Just clearing away the trauma that stops, the trauma that blocks, the trauma that is stuck in some long forgotten past. We may ask, is it this life or past life? First look to this life. See the patterns. bring it to this life first. But past life will show you repeated patterns. And possibly why you chose the family with the ancestral frequencies and stories running in their blood, as lessons for your growth. What past events are you stuck in? And final question! How can you align to your higher self who is clear of all of that, what does she look and feel like? Bringing her close each day.

Five Exercises in Clearing, for Fully Believing & Aligning

Firstly you need to *really* believe that this dream birth is possible!

Returning to the previous discussion about the power of words and truth, let's comb through the dream birth plan and ensure that you can fully believe in it by following these exercises. Working through any negative thoughts, beliefs and emotions, is essential to power up and align into your intention.

Exercise One

Look at what you want and summarise your birth visualisation into clear and precise headings.

For example:

Within

    Feeling relaxed

    Smooth

    Laughter and fun

Without

    In a water birthing pool

    Johnny present, midwives outside

    Quiet, no music at all.

Exercise Two

Now light a candle to invoke a sacred space and connect with you heart. Then from this sacred place of connection, look at each heading and imagine that it is possible by saying *"I believe that … is possible"*. After saying this, sit with it and just feel what your responses might be.

Then write down all the thoughts and feelings (good and bad) that arise from repeating this statement and also include expectations and life situations that help or hinder that particular dream birth quality. Bypass the mind and write from your heart.

At this point, you can also refer to the Tuning In Meditation in Step 4 and, if necessary, keep repeating it to see what your heart feels.

You must tune into all your nagging doubts and state what they are. This is essential part of manifesting your birth. You need to face and release the hidden subconscious blocks. These will be shown to you in sacred space by just sitting with it and asking something to be shown to you. You need to make the time to do this often. It might be things seemingly completely unrelated.

Examples of common doubts could include: your birth partner not being able to support you, your relationship issues, your other children not being safe or looked after or feeling left out, afraid or abandoned, the midwife not being very nice, being unable to support yourself and losing your power, the birthing space options being limited, fear and pain in the birth itself, the cervix not opening, lack of privacy, pelvis not big enough, being judged for making noise, being separated from the baby, not having wishes honoured and respected, dying in labour, or the baby dying in birth, losing control, having intervention or not knowing what to do, being unable to relax... and so on.

Remember, it is good to identify and clear the negatives while you are pregnant so that they won't arise in the birth space.

Make sure you include **all** the negative feelings that you feel hinder your success in achieving what you want.

We are looking to create awareness here, rather than analysis. This means just sitting and being with each challenge or resistance or fear that presents itself, just noticing what arises, where in your body you feel it, what thoughts arise etc. Whilst it is best to use key words rather than filling pages of analysis, if you feel you do want to write lots, that is also fine: follow your intuition.

For example:

Within

Feeling Relaxed –

GOOD...can relax quite easily when I am massaged / John is good at massage. I feel very comfortable with the first stage.

BAD...notice tension in tummy when think about Tommy, should we have a baby sitter? Who? How will that work? Worried about John's work load, will he be able to support me?

Note – I need to tune into where this feeling of tension comes from. It feels familiar...have I felt it before at any other time in my life? Is there an underlying belief here that needs changing? I need to do some releasing energy work on this. What mantra comes to me when I shut my eyes to heal this hurt? Put the request to my Higher Self and listen for the words. I have memory of my own step dad not being able to be there for my mum when she gave birth, its just a sense. I recall feeling this concern of the man not holding the woman when i was about 4.....

Smooth –

GOOD...Really get a sense of what smooth means and that this is possible. Can imagine baby as smooth.

BAD...no bad, I can really tune into smooth and I know that this IS a truth for me.

Without

John present, midwives outside –

GOOD...John and I would birth well together, he helps me relax, and can guard the door!

BAD...Feel anxious John may let midwifes in if they are demanding or that they will need to observe me...Is this the same anxiety as above? The same feeling an underlying cause? Is this about a man being able to hold the container? Again the first time I felt this was aged 4 when.....

Try to get beyond the thoughts into the feelings. Here Christa is noticing her feelings and resistances but trying to approach them with her mind. She needs to drop deeper still to connect to the feeling of being unsafe, and see what that feels like, looks like, what age she was, call in her inner child and directly connect to the inner feeling of being unsafe.

Do this for each heading.

Exercise Three

Let's look at the things that you feel could hinder your birth, your blocks and resistances. Let's try and heal them.

We can do this by changing the feeling internally through inner presence and healing light (within) AND by changing the situation externally through action (without) - using both the inner and the outer, the yin and the yang, to create resolution.

For the rest of this step, you will look into changing your WITHIN and WITHOUT keywords by making adjustments to your external environment, then in the next step you will take a look at *transforming your inner feelings in order to affect your internal environment.*

One by one, go through your list and work out what you can do to change what is hindering your dream birth in the external world. Start an action plan right now to create opportunities without to resolve the hindrances, as well as all the things you could do to create your dream birth.

Write them down as key pointers.

For example:

> Key word - Worried Tommy
> Do I want baby sitters on hand? - could feel at ease
> with Annabel... Phone some Doulas... Speak with neighbours.
> . Could Mum be around? Do I want her around?
> Rely on midwives and John? Speak to midwife...

You need to make opportunities in your life to create what you want. Begin by making some phone calls or whatever you need to do.

Once you have put out what you want to the universe, you do not need to worry about the HOW (let spirit do that), but you still need to create opportunities in a relaxed way.

Do you see the difference? It means you create opportunities but do not hold onto them, just look and create them. You create the opportunities for the universe to make it happen. It might happen (most likely) in ways that never occurred to you.

For example, after our wonderful home birth, Matthew developed bad flu and could not look after me, our toddler and the new baby. No relatives were about as we had asked them to stay away for various reasons. All night long I kept saying to the universe, "I have a babysitter for my toddler and someone to cook. I don't know who or how, it is up to you. Help!" I then let go and trusted it would somehow be okay. In the morning I made three phone calls. The midwife's daughter's friend happened to be a nanny who was free that day. She was there within the hour and ended up coming for nearly two years on and off to help out! She was the right person for us at that time. Not only did I affirm and change my fear into trust by addressing the emotion, I also created the opportunity by making the calls and taking action. This is the yang. But of course I also had some inner yin energy work to do…and this are covered in the next steps -

Exercise Four

Now you have all your negative feelings out, you are en route to your positive birth. But before you proceed to the next step, where you will address your inner feelings, please ensure that you feel you have covered everything: once more comb through quickly with your eyes shut and see if there is anything you might have left out.

Just sit a while once more with the negative worries and hindrances to your birth plan. We will be looking at fear release later, but for now just sit with your feelings and ask **"What is the root of this feeling?"** and write down anything else that could arise.

For example, it might be that your relationship needs healing, or that you are nervous about abandoning your other children. You would then make a note of all your emotions around this.

MIND CHATTER - Worried about Tommy….Why am I worried about him? He is still so small and might not understand what is happening, he might get scared or left alone in the birth.

EMOTION - I feel like I am abandoning him by having another baby. I feel hurt in my heart and my tummy like I can't breathe when I think of him scared in the birth and afterwards when he sees me with another baby. He is very clingy at the moment…

GOING DEEPER - This hurt is the same feeling as my hurt with John. I felt it when I was 4 when dad went away and Joanne was born. I have this belief that one is abandoned when the other is born. I have a belief that this is how it is. I need to change this. What is my mantra for this? Let me tune into this feeling of hurt that I felt as a child myself and ask my Higher Self for the mantra…

INTO SACRED SPACE - I see red roots, i see the fear as a tightening it has a particular shape, i start to pull it out and hold it in my hands, i can feel ti squirming around and I ask ti to show me more, i see an image of something strange, a man slapping a woman, i dont recall this happening, but it is what i am shown. I ask for *more, i am told to take this feeling to clear, so i bring in light into it and feel it clear in the light in my tummy, it transforms into a new shape, and the man is now holding the woman, he is apologising...*

Keep on writing and feeling in, even though it may feel like jargon at first or as if you are making it all up. Eventually you may find that many of the so-called 'fears' are all the same fear and relate to only one or a few inner beliefs or trauma feelings that need addressing. It's fascinating to start to find the root causes!

For example, Veronica had a slight sensation now and again that her baby would get stuck. She recognised this was a fear and instead of ignoring it in the hope that it would go away, she worked through why she felt this fear whilst doing mirror and mantra work and working through deeper issues. By talking to her heart, she related it to blocks around a woman's worth and her body ability to open to the full easily, due to a lack of belief in women's ability and worth from a childhood trauma. She kept imagining her baby gliding out smoothly and easily, and affirmed this daily amongst her other mantras. She eventually got to the point where she really felt that her baby glided smoothly and she knew she had really eliminated that fear (and in the meantime healed a feeling that had affected her in many other ways). Sure enough, in the birth her baby glided out easily and well, exactly as she had affirmed and felt.

Exercise Five

The Holy Grail

Your womb is the Holy Grail. This is the biggest esoteric secret referred to throughout time in mythology, in the great arts and literatures of the ages. The holy grail is the sacred chalice, she is the portal to the Goddess, from here life is born. This is the power of womb, of woman, this is the power of the bride. This is the power fo the birthing woman. This is the sacred way that priestesses live by. The sacred rose of the yoni, the vagina, is the eye portal painted as a gateway in so much art. This is the centre of the symbol the vesica pisces. This is the fish symbol. It also refers direct to the pineal gland.

There are many ways to start working with you womb as grail, as sacred. You can see all the organs of the sacred area as 7 gateways in. You can journey with them and through them. You can work with the rose petals and do blessing ceremonies to honour her. When you are not pregnant, you can do yoni steams if they work for you (not all yonis want this) or work with yoni crystal eggs and look to giving you blood to the earth. Or you can just talk to her. Here are two simple ways to work with chalice that relate directly to this step in finding your power mantras.

1. The Chalice Temple

Imagine your womb is a sacred chalice.
Place one hand on womb and one hand on heart and connect the 2 with deep breaths.
Imagine entering your heart and finding a tunnel and from here you journey through until you reach a beautiful temple or cave. This is you womb portal.
Enter into her and see how she looks.

Imagine you have a paintbrush of light and you go around and paint her fresh and everything the brush touches it turns to light.

Note what things are there that should not be, note any old cords to old relationships that need to be released and dissolved, any old wounds or traumas, messages that are stored here. Are there any strange objects that you need to clear out?

Decorate her and make her beautiful with flowers, light, crystals, colour.

In the centre is an altar, this is your womb altar. You can call in holy mother, or you womb spirit to show herself here. Place the unwanted things in there on the alter and ask the light to transform them into something new and beautiful. This is pure alchemy.

Keep going until you know you are done.

Finally ask for key words and messages to come forth, when you travel back to your heart and through the gateway to waking consciousness, bring them with you.

2. The Cauldron Technique

imagine you hold a beautiful cauldron in the middle of a sacred temple.

Place all unwarned feelings, thoughts, beliefs into the cauldron.

Ask a spiriting to come and then pour in the light form heavens into the cauldron to alchemise all that is there.

As this happens feel it happen in you own body

Let everything transform into something new and beautiful.

When you have the new and beautiful things ask for them to come into words.

See how the cauldron has transformed into a beautiful new vessel and the old within it has become the new, see the new in the new vessel held by mother goddess before you.

Feel this happening within you body.

You can do this in 5 minutes o you can take a whole hour in set sacred ceremonial space.

Step Seven

Realising Your Core Birth Power Mantras

Make two columns.

Note down in the first column the key words about your fears from the previous exercise.

NOW WE ARE GOING WITHIN to address the inner energy core beliefs, emotions and traumas even further.

First you will ask for anything related to come forth, anything at all. Ask for your heart just to speak to you, any age you were, any colour, any emotion, that is a hindrance to your dream, that needs addressing. Sit and say your fear with your eyes closed and as you do so, ask for the core wounding to come.

You will then take the core wounding and hold it and bring the light in and shine it in.

As you do this feel it change shape in your body and healing to take place. You can get help with this if you wish through an energy healer but also do it alone with Goddess, She will bring Her Light in to transform whatever arises.

Then once you feel it start to lift, ask for an affirmation or mantra that addresses it and brings in the new energy feeling of light, to come to you.

When it comes, write it down in the opposite column.

Do this for all your fears/key words from the previous step.

You can draw upon the previous exercises in the previous step to really fine tune and realise these mantras so that they come in direct from within you. From your heart, your womb, your baby, your subconscious, your Higher Self and your spirit guides.

1. Worried about Tommy - Mantra re. Tommy.

He may get scared in the birth -
I feel a need to control Tommy to protect him from when I saw my dad leave aged 6, i feel the fear of dad leaving and how I had to make everything okay and take responsibility for mum and rebecca... bringing this to light......I felt resolution of this story and saw my 6 year old self rise in wholeness...I took time with this and eventually the mantra that came was a deep feeling that he is okay and i saw a blue light within him....

He may be left alone in the birth -

- He will be protected and with someone he loves during the birth and I felt this in the blue light, i have aligned this desire to blue light and felt it become so

I felt like I am abandoning him by having another baby –
- I know and now feel from this blue light and the sunshine that came and filled me that I have enough love for everyone and may love him even better with two!

I felt hurt in my heart and my tummy but this dissolved when i went into the story of when i was 6 –
- I now can feel light and happiness in my heart and tummy. Now I fill with white light and trust.

I could not breathe when I thought of him scared in the birth and afterwards when he sees me with another baby. After this blue light came, that evaporated and I saw all the fear transform in the light to butterflies of freedom freeing us all up into light –
- I now breathe easily and feel the space at ease and with happiness. The vibe around me of safety and warmth in the birth emanates to everyone.

He is very clingy at the moment – I now see and feel him soften as I release this fear and I am working to shift it into the new feeling
- He will be so happy to see his new brother or sister and see only love. He now feels safe and protected and secure.

Conclusion: I see and feel more light now, I can feel him as secure and happy during the birth, and there is someone looking after him who I like. I feel like I can let go of this fear now knowing that he is well. I feel that a new baby will be a delight for us not a threat. I feel release in my heart and tummy as I know all is well.

Fine Tuning your Mantras

From the last 2 steps and the exercises, you now have core mantras that come in direct from sacred space. They are not from your mind, they are yours that you have been given through doing the inner work in sacred space and this gives them huge power.

Say the mantras that come to you via the inner every single day. Play around with the mantras - some may not seem relevant after a few days or some of the words may not sit right and need changing. Keep on noting the energetic vibrations of each affirmation within you.

A word on tenses. Your heart and sacred space will have presented to you mantras in the above exercise that are in the present tense and please keep them that way. The subconscious only recognises positive language, so you need to keep your mantras in the positive tense. For example, if you say to a child "don't jump" or "don't touch the radiator" the body automatically hears the main words, "jump" or "touch radiator". Instead, it could be better to say "let's be still" or "Ow! Radiator hot, keep hands away!".

You can also re-affirm your core power mantras by changing the tense, i.e. from "me" to "you". When writing out some affirmations one day, I recognised that what we want others to do is often what we need to do for ourselves. You may find that what others do to you is exactly related to how you feel about yourself. It is a good idea to bear this in mind when writing mantras and rewrite them or say each one in a different tense.

Take a simple mantra like *"children are good to me"*.
This can be supported by *"I am good to children, I am good to me, all others are good to me, I am good to others"*.
Then it can be changed to *"children are good to you, you are good to children, you are good to yourself, others are good to you, you are good to others"*.

You could also change the "to" to a "for", and see how that changes the feeling and vibration of the mantra.

You may find that your mantras are all related to one inner fear/belief so you may end up amalgamating some of the mantras into one.

Bring light and colour and feeling to your mantras. You can even give them sounds and shapes by drawing them. You can set them to music by imagining a piece of music and asking the light of you mantras to be aligned to that music so that whenever you listen to it you receive the power of your very own core mantra.

Step Eight

Now you can fully believe that you are worthy of it

Who am I to have a dream birth?

You are a child of God.
You are, you exist.

It is, therefore, your birthright.

The *Desiderata* (Max Ehrmann, 1927) states that "*You are a child of God, You have as much right to be here as the stars and trees*". You have as much worth and right to shine as brightly as the stars and grow like the most abundant tree.

Every single human has a unique talent and a unique signature and inner spark of God.

Focus on your 'have' attitude and your worthiness for having your dream birth.

Sit with your hand on your tummy and your other hand on your heart and say this until you feel it:

I am a child of God.

I am worthy of the perfect birth.

It is my birthright.

Please reflect on this simple step for a whole day.

This is all about your worthiness and value.

Now check in and see if you fully believe that this can happen.

In order to manifest, you BELIEVE, and you ALLOW.

Step Nine

Your Birth Power Mantra Sheet

The following exercise is the creation of your birthing mantra sheet.

Take a blank A4 piece of paper. Fold it in half. Look at your beautiful dream birth from Steps One to Six and write it out again to fit one half of A4:

My Beautiful Birth Intention
....

Inside the paper, write out your positive mantras on one entire page.

My Core Birth Power Mantras
....
....

Inside the paper you will then have your birthing mantras to do each day. Outside the paper you will have a clear succinct account of your dream birth. You may have lots of different mantras but when you tune in and write them, you may notice patterns and see that they are related to only a few inner beliefs and emotions and that just a few mantras are enough.

On the other side, on the blank half, condense your mantras down to five key phrases and words and /or write a basic summary of your personal affirmations to read and affirm regularly.

Examples of five key phrases.

Sue's personal mantras were:
1. Angel. Sanctuary. Birth from within.
2. Quiet: Space and time.
3. Nurtured - Nourished by Mother Earth
4. Feel supported and listened to by all present
5. Birth from my power (others are merely there to support my wishes)

Belinda's five key phrases were:
1. tinkly sparkly golden shivers and ripples of waves, joyous ripples of golden
    light
2. deeper deeper

3. floppy muscles soft like jelly
4. golden and white light open cervix and surge baby down
5. angels guiding you

Belinda shortened this further into a summary of just 5 words:
1. light
2. relax
3. surrender
4. all ok
5. happy

You can use the visualisations in this book to include the names of guides and spirit midwives in your key phrases.

Carry this paper with you. Keep it with you all day long, look at it first thing in the morning and last thing at night and before you sit quietly in the day.

This piece of paper is your personal Birthing Power Mantra Sheet.

As you read Part Two, you will rewrite this several times - the more the better as you may add to or remove things as new things emerge and others are resolved. More will most certainly arise. As you peel off one layer, a new one may reveal itself. You may find that patterns arise and you spot a link between them or trace the patterns back to something entirely different. In this case, you can go back to the simple inner clearing work, or if you need to then you can take further action to support your affirmations and get support for inner energy work – see a healer, do some emotional freedom techniques, Reiki, find some flower essences. Whatever you are drawn to. You will learn more about this in Part Two.

You can record your mantras and your dream birth plan into your phone and listen to them regularly. As suggested already you can also set them to music. Let your birthing partner read the plan when you have finished so that they can share and support your needs and help create it by also imagining it for you. In the birth they can help to remind you of your plans. You could ask them to read them regularly so that you become comfortable with their voice in the birth. Their voice, saying that key phrase, will become a signal for relaxation for you.

Make time to create a set space to focus on this every day. Take your time and really imagine it happening, see yourself in that light and healthy space.

Each time you sit in your set space, look at the three statements discussed in this chapter, and say:

"I believe that my dream birth of ... is possible. I fully believe it and I fully believe that I am worthy of it."

Read out your dream birth. Then go through your positive affirmations and say each one aloud.

End each and every affirmation with the words:

"for the highest good of all concerned, so be it and so it is"

Then finally:

"and now I let it go".

Example Birthing Mantras

You have created your own unique power mantras direct from your subconscious already. They come from the quantum field. Now that you have <u>your very own</u> power mantras, the following are examples of birthing mantras for inspiration. You can also look at these and other mantras because one or 2 may leap out and really sing to your heart or womb. So run your finger down the list and see which ones leap out to add to you very pose core power ones and hold them next to you and feel a yes or no response form you subconscious within as you say or touch them.

So some might really speak to you, whilst others may not. Only use those which resonate within and always tune in for your unique body guidance.

These can be used anytime. There are further examples in Part Three of mantras that you can use from week thirty two when the baby has reached the right size. You can reflect on how to turn your mantras into prayer in Part Two.

Remember that you can use mantras spoken out loud or silently or sung, during pregnancy, the birth and whilst parenting as a quick device for reaching stillness. However you decide to affirm, picture the affirmations as you say them.

Keep the mantras in the present tense. For example, if you say "I want..." all the universe will do is mirror your want. You need to say "I now have..." If this seems like a lie at first, keep trying with it anyway. Notice your disbelief and keep on saying it until you can believe it. **It is the emotion behind the affirmation that gives it power and that sets the vibration of the words to resonate out into the universe.**

Remember to change the tenses from past to present and from "I" to "you" as you read each one and to keep them in the positive tense.

- *I give up birthing to my body and baby*
- *Birth is a joyful experience!*
- *We are safe and all is well*
- *I birth easily and well*
- *I am relaxed*
- *I surrender to the LIGHT and I trust*
- *I give over to my baby and body*
- *I am supported by the Light, I feel held*
- *My body is strong and births my baby easily*
- *My baby glides easily through my pelvis*
- *Birth is a dance, I move and sway the dance*

- *I connect to all other birthing women who are birthing right now*
- *I am linked to my birth, my mother's birth and my mother's mother's birth in this moment!*
- *I handle each surge and find stillness within the sensation with my breath*
- *I have the energy and stamina to birth my baby*
- *I give over to GOD and Divine Guidance*
- *I am in touch with my inner intuition*
- *My inner presence is guiding and providing all that I need*
- *I am in tune with my body*
- *I go out of my head and enter my body: relaxed, relaxed, relaxed!*
- *I have surrendered*
- *I am happy*
- *I am at ease*
- *I feel birth smoothly and comfortably*
- *My baby glides out easily like a dolphin*
- *My womb is full of light*
- *My body and my baby know what to do*
- *My partner supports me easily and well*
- *I feel connected to myself, my baby, my body and my partner*
- *I am protected and safe*
- *My womb is filled with womb light!*
- *I am the source*
- *I am worthy of an amazing birth*
- *I love and honour myself*
- *Everything is rolling just as it is meant to. I feel the magic of this birth as everything that I need is instantly provided for*
- *I enjoy the birthing sensations*
- *I am able to protect my space as my baby enters this world*
- *I welcome my baby with loving arms and maintain a sacred space*
- *I am looked after and everything happens just as it should do for my highest good*
- *I open up easily and well*
- *I am able to talk with my body with love during birthing*
- *I enjoy a sense of grace during birth*
- *I keep my arms, legs, pelvic floor, and face totally relaxed*
- *As I open up easily, I sense beautiful ripples in my muscles. This is as it should be: enjoyable and in the fullness of my power as woman*
- *My only responsibility is to control my mind. My body will birth my baby safely and efficiently into my loving arms*
- *I am open to follow the signs whatever they might be and I am in tune with God and my intuition, beyond and regardless of what my mind might impose on me.*
- *Praise God for the light within me – God is my source*
- *All evil vanishes from life for him who keeps the sun in his heart!*
- *My children are divinely protected and surrounded by love*
- *I am surrounded by white light*

The Power Birthing Mantra

Focus on a Divine Mother image that calls you and place it on your altar to watch over you.
Every time you look at Her, say 3 times - "I surrender to Light".
Follow this by saying 3 times - "I am Light".
Do this in the birth space too.

Birth-specific Mantras
When considering birth-specific mantras regarding the great opening of your cervix, leave these until nearer the birth time. More on this later in the book.

- *I open and open wide knowing I am safe to do so*
- *I see my cervix opening wide with each wave*
- *My cervix opens more and more each day with ease and with love.*

Birth Mantras from 32 Weeks
These are in Part Three

Completion
You might like to complete with a mantra like this, or in your own words *"for the highest good of all concerned in all directions of time. So be it and so it is"*
Then remember to act "as if" and BELIEVE…
really feel the energy and intent of the words.
Let it go to Goddess now in beautiful eternal flow of Light.

Ancient Mantras (Seed Mantras)

You may also wish to explore some mantras from other cultures and traditions that can be very powerful. There are a few mantras here from different spiritual traditions/languages. Please look up and listen to the correct pronunciations on You Tube. I suggest you also buy some Kundalini Yoga mantra music from Spirit Voyage and chant along. Seed mantras mean that the sounds of the words themselves have a vibrational quality that is one with God and can shift the entire energy in a room instantly to one of calm and equilibrium.

1. Om Mani Padme Hum
(God is the jewel in the centre of the lotus made manifest in my heart). This is a Buddhist Sanskrit Mantra used in Tibet.

2. Om Bhuur-Bhuvar Svah
Tat-Savitur-Varennyam
Bhargo Devasya Dhiimahi
Dhiyo Yo Nah Pracodayaat
The Devi Gayatri Mantra, cited in Hindu texts such as Bhagavhad Gita. Some say it is 6000 years old!

3. Om Namah Shivaya
Hindu Mantra, also used in Shaivism. Its translation is "adoration to Shiva, preceded by the mystical syllable 'Aum'. Babaji, the great Indian Sage, says "This Om Namah Shivaya is like nectar; feed everyone with this nectar. Sri Mahaprabhuji wishes that all words would disappear from this world, except for three - Om Namah Shivaya. This is the original mantra. When Primordial Energy first appeared, the first mantra that She uttered from Her Holy mouth was Om Namah Shivaya". Babaji also said that "The energy of Om Namah Shivaya shall destroy all contradictory energies of hydrogen and atom bombs and will protect you. There are proofs in the scriptures, that it was the great Gautama Rishi who

created the atom energy, and he has said clearly that the only thing that can conquer the atom energy is the Om Namah Shivaya mantra, by itself."

4. Aum or Om

"The goal which all the Vedas declare, which all austerities aim at, and which men desire when they lead the life of continence ... is Om. This syllable Om is indeed Brahman. Whosoever knows this syllable obtains all that he desires. This is the best support; this is the highest support. Whosoever knows this support is adored in the world of Brahma."~ Katha Upanishad I. This single syllable is of paramount importance within Hinduism.

6. The Kirtan Kriya

This meditation comes from Kundalini Yoga practise. The following is taken from *The Aquarian Teacher*, byYogi Bhajan, p425.

"The meditation brings a total mental balance to the individual psyche. Vibrating on each fingertip alternates the electrical polarities. The index and ring fingers are electrically negative, relative to the other fingers. This causes a balance in the elector magnetic projection of the aura. Practicing this meditation is both a science and an art. It is an art in the way it moulds consciousness and in the refinement of sensation and insight it produces. It is a science in the tested certainty of the results each technique produces. Meditations have coded actions to their reactions in the psyche. But because Kirtan Kriya is effective and exact, it can also lead to problems if not done properly....Yogi Bhajan said at Winter Solstice 1972 that a person who wears pure white and meditates on this sound current for 2 1/2 hours a day for one year, will know the unknowable and see the unseeable. Through this constant practise, the mind awakens to the infinite capacity of the soul for sacrifice, service, and creation."

Time Required - 31 minutes (or less but keep to time proportions as below).
Try this for 40 days.

Tune In -   Always tune in with the Adi Mantra ONG NAMO GURU DEV NAMO. This always precedes Kundalini Yoga practice, tuning one in to the higher self. Ong is "Infinite Creative energy in manifestation and activity" (Om or Aum is God absolute and unmanifested), Namo is "reverent greetings' implying humility, Guru means "teacher or wisdom", Dev means "Divine or of God" and Namo reaffirms humility and reverence. In all it means, "I call upon Divine Wisdom".

Protection Mantra - You can continue tuning in with the Mangala Charn Mantra mantra, AD GURAY NAMEH, JUGAD GURAY NAMEH, SAT GURAY NAMEH, SIRI GURU DEVAY NAMEH, which is chanted for protection. It surrounds the magnetic field with protective light, and means "I bow to the primal Guru (guiding consciousness who takes us to God-Realization), I bow to wisdom through the ages, I bow to True Wisdom, I bow to the great, unseen wisdom."

Sit - Sit straight in Easy Pose (cross legged).
Eye Position - Meditate at the Brow Point (Third Eye)

Mantra - Produce the five primal sounds (panj shabd): S,T,N,M,A in the original word form:
SAA - infinity, cosmos, beginning
TAA - Life, existence

NAA - Death, change. transformation
MAA - Rebirth
Each repetition of the entire mantra takes 3-4 seconds.
This is the cycle of creation. From the infinite comes life and individual existence.
From life comes death or change.
From death comes the rebirth of consciousness to the joy of the infinite through which compassion leads back to life.

Mudra - This mantra can be done in many different mudras. Most common is to begin in Gyan Mudra. The elbows are straight while chanting (hands rest on knees), and the mudra changes as each fingertip touches in turn the tip of the thumb with firm pressure.
On Saa, touch the first (Jupiter) finger
On Taa, touch the second (Saturn) finger
On Naa. touch the third (Sun) finger
On Maa, touch the fourth (Mercury) finger

Chant in three languages of consciousness:
Human: normal or loud voice (the world)
Lovers: strong whisper (longing to belong)
Divine: mentally; silent (infinity)

Time - Begin the Kriya in a normal voice for **5 minutes**; then whisper for **5 minutes;** then go deep into the sound, vibrating silently for **10 minutes**. Then come back to a whisper for **5 minutes**, then aloud for **5 minutes**. The duration of the meditation may vary, as long as the proportion of the loud, whisper, silent, whisper, loud is maintained.

To End - This sequence will take 30 minutes. Follow with one minute of silent prayer. Then inhale, exhale. Stretch the spine, with hands up as far as possible, spread the fingers wide, take several deep breaths. Relax.

Checkpoint - If during the silent part of the meditation, the mind wanders uncontrollably, go back to a whisper, to a loud voice, and back into silence. Do this as often as you need to. Some people may experience headaches from practising Kirtan Kriya. The most common reason for this is improper circulation of prana in the solar centres. To avoid or correct this problem, meditate on the primal sounds in the "L" form. This means there is a constant inflow of cosmic energy into the solar centre or Tenth Gate. Imagine the energy of each sound moving through the crown chakra, and out through the Third Eye Point as it is projected to Infinity. This energy flow follows the energy pathways called the Golden Cord - the connection between pineal and pituitary glands. You may also want to try covering the head with a natural fibre (white) cloth.

Tune Out - Always end any Kundalini Yoga practise by Tuning out. Sing the Long Time Sun then chant Sat Nam 3 times, Saaat for a count of 15 and Nam for a count of 3, with hands in prayer pose.

Long Time Sun - May the long time Sun shine upon you, all love surround you and the Pure Light within you, guide your way on, guide your way on (repeat).

NOTE - THE KIRTAN KRIYA IS NOT INTENDED TO BE A SUBSTITUTE FOR PROFESSIONAL MEDICAL ADVICE, DIAGNOSIS OR TREATMENT.

The Love Mantras

Open your heart by repeating these mantras whilst in meditation in your sacred space, on waking, or before sleep. Repeat for anything from 3 to 11 minutes.

I am Love Mantra
I am love, and so are you
You are love, and so am I
We are love, we are love
I am love, I love you
You love me, I love myself, you love yourself
I love the world , the world loves me
I love everyone, everyone loves me
I am loved, you are loved, we are loved
And we are love
I see love in you, you see love in me
We are love and we are one love
You are me and I am you
We are love, I am love
You are love, we are love
I am love
Love
I am
Love

The Love Peace Light Universal Prayer
Love before me
Love behind me
Love at my left
Love at my right
Love above me
Love below me
Love in me
Love in my surroundings
Love to all
Love to the universe

Repeat the above prayer with the word "Peace" and then with the word "Light".
You can end by inhaling love, holding peace and exhaling light.

Step Ten

Allowing

Mantra of Emotion

Your final exercise is to evoke the mantra of emotion without words: drop the words and just be with and feel the positive emotion. The mantras are just words in your head. The feeling is real. Sometimes it is necessary to chant mantras. Then some days, there are too many words, sometimes too many mantras.

The mantra of emotion is just about being in the space and feeling still and feeling beauty and feeling easy birth. Feel the mantra. Feel the feeling. Use the mantra, use the words to release any pain and tune into a positive trance state. Then drop the words and be in this state. Evoke a feeling and keep it with you. This is the state you need to birth from. Use mantra to create it then release the words completely.

So as you say the positive mantras, you feel the words. After lots of practise saying the words in your personal space, eventually when you sit down you will not need to say the words and can just feel. Then whenever you remember, just return to this feeling. Next time you suddenly start to feel bad or ugly, just tune into the feeling of being beautiful. As well as diving into the subconscious to target and clear the feeling of ugly, tuning into the feeling of being beautiful can also have great power. We work in balance with shadow work and uplift, making sure both are in balance. We do not do too much shadow work, but nor do we ignore shadow and constantly live in denial on the surface. you get the balance right.

And so when doing uplift work, just by tuning into the feeling of being beautiful, you will be beautiful immediately and others will perceive you as beautiful. Likewise, just by tuning into easy birth, you will have an easy birth and others will perceive you as having an easy birth and you will start to attract the experiences that initiate easy birth. It can sometimes be that easy too.

So, start to leave the words and just tune into the positive feeling.

Evoke a feeling and keep it with you. Just be in the space, feeling still and feeling your breath and just keep on being with your meditation and feel the mantra. Use your imagination:

I feel rich - feel this feeling of seeing money pouring towards you
I feel an easy birth - feel this feeling of a flowing and easy birth.

(if you continue to feel resistance then return to step 6 & 7 to do the shadow release of any inner feelings or subconscious survival programs that need to be cleared that might be running to prevent this feeling from anchoring in deeper)

Use an image to help with this - I SEE money coming towards me, I SEE a baby gliding out healthy, well and easily. Keep the image with the feeling and the words.

Find a crystal, ring, necklace or anything to hold that represents your key feeling and keep this with you during your pregnancy and birth.

Letting Go = Allowing it to Happen

There comes a point you have to surrender all to Goddess and trust in her that this will happen and is happening and have absolutely belief your birth intention is manifesting. You can do a ceremony in any way you wish before a beautiful birth altar and candle to speak your mantras and intention and give it to goddess with absolute faith. when you set this up as ritual this gives it great power. The prayer of the birthing mother is always heard. Through the rest of this book you will dive deeper into this.

"When you know your ship is unsinkable, you don't worry about icebergs or lifeboats"

The beauty of creating a set space for your birth work is that, afterwards, you can let it go and carry on with your day knowing that the work has been done. Even if you keep saying your mantras through the day, you have done the manifestation already in your set space.

Letting go is very important. The moment you let go of something, it happens. How many times have you thought, "I wish he/she would call" and carried that NEED around during the day, niggling away. The moment you let go of the NEED and move on and do not mind (when the tension has gone) then they will call.

*"By letting it go all gets done
The world is won by those who let it go.
But when you try and try
The word is then beyond the winning"*
Tao Te Ching

Believe it AS IF this is how it is going to be. Know that this is how it is going to be.

I was watching some birds in a tree a few days ago. They did not use their minds. They just hung out on a branch. Then following the rhythm of nature, no thought, they just got up and went to another. And hung out again. Then again, up they went, all at the same time this time. How did they all know that was the moment? They didn't. They're just surfing the wave of natures. The energy of the tree...The flow around them. And again, whoosh, they all moved on. Then still. Hanging out. Suddenly one flies to the ground, picks a worm and returns. How did it know? How did it catch the worm? It was in the vibe. In tune. If you are in tune, you catch the worm. If you are in tune, you are in the right place at the right time for you and your baby.

Note down any negative thoughts or feelings that arise and keep releasing them so that you can fully believe. . If you order something, you have to then LET GO and trust that it is. So let these negative feelings go and believe.

Then start making steps towards creating the opportunities in the external world, if you feel guided to do so, but let go, let your dream go to the universe and follow the instincts you receive, let the universe guide the HOW.

There is an old story that perfectly describes the secret of manifestation: A man once went with a tribesman to a power spot to pray for rain. Expecting a ceremony, the man was very surprised when, after the tribesman had been standing still for just 5 minutes, he then turned to leave. "Is that it?" The man exclaimed "You have not done anything yet?!" The tribesman smiled and replied "But I have. All I did was feel the rain: I just feel it raining…If I pray for rain I am only putting out my lack and NEED, but standing here like this I can feel it!"

This is why so many prayers do not get answered: we put out our NEED, our lack, instead of affirming the feeling of having what we want and assuming we have it. Feel a wonderful birth and it will be yours, feel your children happy and they will be.

So learn this now: that the great secret of manifestation is to feel what you want AS IF it already exists.

Therefore act AS IF.

Eradicate any thoughts, feelings, people, situations that do not support your dream birth from now on. We will talk about how to get support in this from your birthing partner later on. You may find you have to avoid certain people or situations for a while. This is fine, you could tell people that you are going to lie low for a while and rest and even phone people to announce this.

When we do what we want, we can be free. Doing what we feel we *have* to do or *should* do leads to war, destruction and unhappiness for everyone. It does not allow anyone to be free. Wherever you see the word "should", replace it with the word "could" and see what effect this simple action has on your life. If you are following your calling and doing your "thing" then you will be at ease with everything that happens. Be a leader, not a follower. If you are worried about being others talking about you, then look at where the people who do this are. Do you want to be in their reality of lack or in one of power?

From now on, make a conscious decision to only entertain positive birth stories and expectations that support your dream birth. There is a protection meditation in Part Two to help with this.

From now on act 'as if'.

To start with, just for today, try and believe that it is possible, even if you can't see how. Imagine it has happened - HOW DOES IT FEEL? Start to walk and talks, as if it is so. Start to speak with language as if it is so. Do not allow in any body, event, language, situation, that feels or thinks otherwise. Have clear boundaries and be aware.

You now know that this is what you REALLY want, so let's make it happen.

Anything is possible, but you need to be clear about what you want and you need to believe one hundred percent.

Don't worry too much about the how, just believe and then follow your instincts on the steps to take. Let the universe do the HOW - as you of course also go about your own inspired action plan to create opportunities, by following the energy – only see people and go places that feel like they "hum", which shine in some way.

You decide what your birth will be.

A. Where is your mind at the moment and what do you believe at the moment?
B. What would you be and what would you have in an illusory world?

The rest of this book is about making that leap from A to B.

Only you can do it, no one else can do it for you. Take up your power now and don't hide behind blaming situations and people.

You can create this birth.

How does that make you feel?

Now you have reached the end of Part One, you will be clear how to find the right mantras applicable for you and your birth.

In Part Two, you will learn more about the importance of clear thoughts and emotions when working with Mantra and how mantras work, before going on to explore further Intuitive Birthing techniques. As you read through Part Two, your mantras may keep changing and you can keep revisiting Part One as much as you like, to access your subconscious and target any trauma or blocks.

Summary of the Themes looked at in the Ten Steps

Feeling into your Birth Intention - is it an inner 'need' or a 'heart inspiration'? Are you imposing upon or allowing? Do you feel aligned to this in you life right now and if not, what is not in alignment?

Connecting to you heart for her desire and messages

Feeling any niggles or resistance. Where do you feel this? When did you first ever feel this feeling? Ask your intuition and subconscious and spirit guides to show you any messages and bring the Light into it for healing and resolution on the inner

Writing it down using key words and writing from the heart

Feeling into any fear, taking it to sacred space, to the subconscious and to the light for guidance, messages, more information and resolution

Drawing pictures and finding key images that summarise this resolution and the new good feeling from the release

From this, creating key words and colours and symbols that summarise this good feeling

Spending time feeling these, allowing them to become manifest. Asking for more words and emotions to flow in to Light.

Repeating these words as they become your Birth Power Mantras, both feeling and imagining throughout the day (also known as the practise of Japa).

Carry a symbol of this mantra to remind you to feel this feeling at all times e.g. a crystal, necklace or ring, or even set to music.

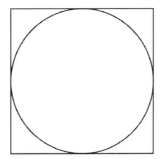

Part Two

Intuitive Birthing Techniques

1 - Clear Thoughts

"We are what we think. All that we are arises with our thoughts. With our thoughts we make the world. Your worst enemy cannot harm you as much as your own mind, unguarded. But once mastered, no one can help you as much. Mind is the forerunner of all states. Mind is chief; Mind-made are those states. The person who suffers most in this world is the person who has many wrong perceptions…and many of our Perceptions are erroneous." (the opening of the Dhammapada).

"Whatever the mind of man can conceive, it can achieve"
W. Clement Stone

"You are sending energy to wherever your thoughts are right now"
Martin Brofman

"Imagination is everything. It is the preview of life's coming attractions."
Albert Einstein

"What you expect and believe is what you experience"
The law of cause and effect.

"You create your own universe as you go along"
Winston Churchill

"Imagination is the queen of truth, and possibility is one of the regions of truth. She is positively akin to infinity."
Baudelaire

"A strong, clear thought with emotion attached to it will precipitate into the astral plane and become clothed in astral matter."
Djwhal Khul channelled through Violet Starre

"All that we are is a result of what we have thought"
Buddha

Descarte's expression "I think therefore I am" could be, instead, "*What* I think is *what* I am".

"All thoughts which have been emotionalised (given feeling) and mixed with faith, begin immediately to translate themselves into their physical equivalent or counterpart"
Think and Grow Rich by Napoleon Hill

*"In your own lives always look forward, anticipate good. By anticipating good, by anticipating blessings and happiness, you are actually drawing those to you; you are creating through your imagination. Imagination is part of the psychic gift implanted in man's soul. Therefore, we say to you from Spirit, use your heavenly imagination, imagine yourself in a state of perfect health, imagine yourself in a state of perfect harmony. If your conditions are harmonious see them becoming smoother, better. Disciplined imagination is the key to creation. Perhaps you are unaware that whenever you think negatively you are actually creating negative conditions for yourself. To create positive good, you must always think positively. If you do this habitually you will clear the mists which gather round you - mists in your own soul, mists in your mind....We cannot impress upon you too strongly to think always in terms of progress, of happiness and of achievement; and you will become healthier and happier. This is our special message for you as you stand at the beginning of a new year. For as you **imagine** your conditions, so you are setting into operation the machinery which will bring about the very picture you hold in your mind. As you **think** light, as you **think** good, you will become a creator, with God, of a beautiful world, a beautiful humanity"*
The Way Of The Sun, White Eagle.

The Power of Thought and Word

To manifest your sacred birth, it is essential that any mental chatter around this topic is brought to awareness, that core beliefs are shown, and that emotions are tuned into.

Your thoughts form your words.
Your words form your deeds and actions.
Your deeds and actions form your habits.
Your habits form your character.
Your character forms your world through friends, events and life choices.

Practising the Mirror Concept

The quickest way to have clear thoughts is by practising the meditation and mantra techniques in Part One. Then you can tune into the underlying belief patterns or emotions resonating within you and see what needs changing. As you do this you will notice more and more the mirror:

*Everything that is happening for you right now
inside you is happening on the outside.
And everything that is happening for you right now
in the outside world is happening within you.*

This universal understanding is called mirror work, and it is a brilliant way of learning what is going on for you and releasing it. If the world is a mirror, then every event, person or situation is a mirror for what is happening inside of you. By being aware of this and taking this awareness into everyday life – at the shops, on the phone etc, you can see what is happening for you inside.

Every single thing is a reflection of the inner energy patterns that you vibrate
Like attracts like
Fear attaches to fear within
Love attaches to love within

You are now to use this understanding to change your inner energy vibration to vibrate with one of sacred birth. And if you want to attract your sacred birth, you must do the inner work to clear any traumatic thoughts, beliefs or emotions that you might be vibrating that are not resonant with sacred birthing. To attract abundance, you must BE abundance within.

When you have a healing, whatever happens in that space is a reflection of the healing process: if the phone rings, note what was happening for you when the phone rang and see what that reflects, it will be directly linked to the treatment. Life is like this. There are no coincidences, no conversations we overhear that do not symbolise something.

For example, Georgia went to a yoga class and the car parking space was very tight, although she just fitted in. When she went in to the class, the space left for her was in the corner and very small. She started to realise that a pattern of small, tight spaces was emerging and decided to look within to see what was small and tight inside of her.

You create everything that happens for you from your own internal space. If you like people, people will like you. If you feel lack in some way, then lack will be shown to you in some way. If you gossip about people, they will gossip about you. Whatever you feel about birth will also be mirrored back to you during your pregnancy in the people and events that you draw to you.

Every thing is about energy.

Remember, there are no accidents in life. Accidents are events that we attract to us to reflect our internal emotional states, and to learn from. Many great things arise from accidents.

Again, try not to get caught up on the analytical side of things. One could dwell on what every event or situation represents, or one could just be aware of it.

So if you note a situation – for example, you are attracting lots of angry people, you could firstly note "ok so I have anger issues around me". Then instead of analysing what/why/whose fault it is, instead release the anger through fear/tension release on the inner through inner energy work, and that will bring in the exact medicine and positive state of calm and peace. Just be with it and sit with it and ask for the message to arise and trust what is shown.

You can also work very simply. if you want to attract something on the outside, for example your sacred birth, then you can breathe and affirm that "I now feel the sacred birth flowing" and imagine sacred birth as a vibration, a colour for example, being drawn in towards you and all around you. Breathe in the energy of sacred birth and feel it. Breathe in a beautiful healthy birth and feel it.

The Power of Words Exercise

Hypnosis is based on this understanding of the power of the mind on our bodies and events. It recognises that by changing our inner thoughts and beliefs, we can change what happens to us or our health. Hypnosis is a powerful tool in birthing. Hypnosis is based on the understanding that the subconscious only recognises positives. Therefore, hypnosis only uses positive terminology. i.e. "I feel really happy" as opposed to "I no longer feel sad".

It is so interesting how a lot of birthing language in our culture is negative.

Close your eyes and try saying some of the various words below, then notice the effect of them on your body. Which words make you feel empowered or more open, or more tense? Notice the vibrations of the words, and start to choose empowering words in everyday situations. Notice how often you choose negative language.

Birthing Word	**Alternate Suggestion**
Labour (implicates the belief system that birth is hard work)	Birthing or birthing process
Effacing / dilating	Thinning / opening
Contraction	Surge or wave
Due date (implies that the date is exact and does not allow for flow, putting pressure on the birthing parents)	Birth time
Pain	Sensation or description of sensation
Waters break (sounds hard, like an accident or a problem)	Membranes release
Baby delivered ("She delivered this baby" also gives the power to another, it is always you who births, whoever may help)	Baby born
Pushing (sounds forced, not relaxed)	Breathing down, birth breath
Complications (nothing is ever wrong or complicated, keep in the flow)	Special circumstances
Miscarriage (implies the woman did not carry well enough)	Loss

Primips/multips	First/Second time mother
Fetus	Preborn/Unborn baby
Catch the baby	Receive the baby

There are many words like this, not just within the pregnancy and birthing language, and it is important that you become aware of your words when talking, and recognise when you and others use these words.

You need to live your truth especially when out and about in the world, not just at home in the bedroom when you are alone. If one moment you are meditating and then the next not living that stillness, you can gently become aware of more consciously living that truth outside the home, making it real.

You can do this with language. As you change your language form victimhood to a more empowered language, become aware of the energetic shifts within.

For example,
◦ changing the word "*should*" for "*could*"
◦ changing the phrase "*I am sorry*" for "*thank you for your patience*"
◦ changing the word "*if*" to "*when*"

See what else you could change and be aware as you talk of limiting words that you may use.

As you become more aware of your language and the subjects that you choose to talk about, you will surprise yourself. You may even find your friends start to shift as you become more conscious of your words. For example, you may notice how you discuss other people with certain friends, and when you don't participate in this they may not be able to relate to you - or alternatively they may shift too.

Feeling deep into your heart and then speaking the words of truth from there is a big exercise and one that many people find difficult in today's culture with its class social structures and expectations/obligations. It is a bigger exercise than it may at first seem. Actually, it is a lifetime's practise to recognise and to speak our truth. Our culture does not recognise the value of being honest within ourselves and most people tell white lies constantly as a way of not hurting others or because they are afraid of the consequences. It is when one has practised speaking truth for a long time that words actually take on power. For example an Indian sage who has practised speaking truth might say "be healed!" and healing will instantly occur.

The power of words is exceptional. Words can be blessings. Words can heal. Words are spoken thought forms. All words are mantras. Babaji, the great Indian sage and guru said to be the incarnation of Shiva himself, said many times that mantra is stronger than the atom bomb! . . . . . .

We need to be exceptionally aware of our thoughts and words. Being thought aware in every day life is hard. We can do this by tuning into our emotions to see where they are. If our thoughts are in accordance with our Higher Self then we will feel good. If not, we need to change our thoughts or our environment. Do not repress nasty thoughts, simply release them through fear without beating yourself up for having them. You are human after all.

"One should not hurt others even by words. One must not speak even an unpleasant thought unnecessarily. By indulging in rude words, one's nature becomes coarse. One's sensibility is lost if one has not control over one's speech."
The Holy Mother – Sri Saradamani Devi.

It is said that masters and gurus can heal people with words alone. There are many tales of Indian gurus using this ability. An example of this might also be the guru Jeshua Ben Joseph, known in new age circles as Sananda and known by Christians as Jesus (who became a channel for Christ Light), a master who used the vibrations of energy to communicate his words. A boy called James who sees vibration energy under regression, describes what his words look like in the book The Power of The Magdalene by Stuart Wilson and Joanna Prentis: *"I can't hear what the speaker is saying…the Light is all around his head, like a rose colour, and they're receiving colour from him"..* This book later describes how *"the vibration of the words themselves can heal at a deep level, and can release blockages deep within us…"*

"I will never forget a day once many years ago when I was a student… I was so cross with my housemate and I was incessantly raging about him with almost venom to my friend, and then a few hours later he returned with a black eye. A bungee cord had sprung back and hit him in the face at almost the exact time I was ranting and raging. When I saw him it was very strange and it seemed absolutely clear to me that I had caused this to happen. It is hard to explain, it was just apparent. In that moment I learnt the power of words."
Matilda, counsellor.

The power of words in the actual birth space cannot be underestimated. Words are directly related to energy and inner feeling. You can change the energy and heal the feeling by targeting the inner root trauma and this inner work is essential, and yet consciously becoming aware and changing your words does have a great affect too. Your body does what it is told!

"I was in Edinburgh, Scotland, addressing an audience of midwives and mothers. I had just related the story about my friend whose cervix had opened when she wished aloud that it would. A woman in the back of the meeting hall caught my attention with her animated facial expression as she listened to this story. She wanted to talk about her experience during labour with her first baby. She had been sitting on her bed in the first stage of labour (during which the cervix is opening), encircled in her husband's arms. He whispered in her ear "You're marvellous!" and she was sure she felt her cervix open when she heard his words.
"Please say that again!" she told him.
He repeated the words and again she felt her cervix open.
"I know you're going to think I'm crazy," she said, addressing both him and her midwife, "but would you keep saying that?"
Her husband, joined by her midwife, kept up the chant. Soon her cervix was completely dilated, and she pushed her baby out."
Ina May Gaskin, Ina May's Guide to Childbirth

Similarly, be careful what you take on when listening to others. For example, when I was at a yoga class, the yoga teacher decided to specialise in breaching techniques to help a mother with a breached baby, but whilst doing them I felt like I was just tuning into that energy of carrying a breached baby when I wasn't, so I stopped. (There is nothing "wrong" with a breach baby, but it was not my truth and I didn't want it to become my truth).

Whether you choose to avoid talking about it or to explain to people what you are doing is up to you. Some people may not understand and other people may be really open to these ideas. Now is not the time to change the world, now is the time to birth your baby happily and well, to look after yourself. Therefore, do some clear healthy boundary exercises, and do not take on board other people's language and ideas or try and convince others who do not understand your approach.

Thinking Further about Birthing Beliefs

Once you start being aware of the power of words and birthing words used in our culture, it will lead to the ultimate questioning of birthing beliefs within our culture, since words are based on internal beliefs. The more you tune in to say mantras, the more your deep inner beliefs that are traumas and blocks may arise to be looked at, which is great as then you can transform them into healing and into positive internal beliefs.

Start to ask yourself things like:

○ Does birth really have to be painful and hard work?
○ Do breach babies mean you need a caesarean?
○ Does being five days overdue mean you need to be induced? (More about the hidden dangers of induction methods later)
○ Do we need to lie on our backs to birth? (This is an idea that was introduced to make it easier for doctors to see what was happening and to have easy access, but for women it actually inhibits the process of opening up for the baby to come out smoothly).
○ Does the cord need to be cut immediately?
○ Do you have to have strangers present in your birthing space?

There are many, many more…

Whatever anyone says, including medical people, you need to evaluate, research and feel for yourself. Question everything. The medical system is often based on the belief system that mind and body are separate and that spirit does not exist. There are health and safety regulations and boxes to tick that are part of a system set up without individual needs in mind or awareness of the impact and importance of emotional welfare on whole body health and well being.

2 Clear Emotions

We have talked about the power of thought and words.

Your emotions are behind every single thought. The power of a word comes from the emotion, the feeling, behind it. One word can change its energy by the emotion directed through it. Is it a word that comes form inspired feeling, or from a trauma feeling?

Your feelings affect your beliefs and attitudes, thoughts, behaviour, actions, life circumstances, accidents and events.

Your emotions tell you where you are right now and if something is right or needs healing. If you are connected and well then you feel good.

Your emotions have value. Get to know them, get to know if they are false ones based in trauma or pain reaction, which we all have, or genuine ones guiding you what is right for you and genuinely feels good. A yearning for chocolate might feel good in the moment but you feel the knowing it is sugar addiction, or on the other hand you might feel the knowing it is a healthy pleasure. You know, by intuition, whether it is a false trauma desire or a genuine heart desire. You don't want to do something? Is it a resistance to something that you know is right for you or is it a genuine knowing that it is not right. Only you know by self knowing, self listening and giving value to all you feel to speak to you.

Your emotions cause either tension or relaxation. If you deeply believe and feel that birthing is pleasurable and easy, and allow yourself to get into that space, then you will be relaxed. If you are relaxed, you will hear and respond to your instincts and body signals and you will create your pleasurable and easy birth.

Your emotions can be buried so deeply that sometimes you are not even aware of many of them. Some emotions will have been there since the time of conception, picked up from our parents, siblings or life events.

If You have a Dream, then Follow its Light

"Don't worry because you make yourself small by worrying, by being afraid. Expand. Trust in the infinity of God. The infinity of God shall come through you."
Yogi Bhajan

Many people dismiss negativity, knowing the importance of focusing on the positive. However, dismissing can repress certain feelings without resolving them, so the negative emotion is still there and is still being recreated in experiences and body health. It is positive to connect to negative emotion so that you resolve and face it, and can shine Light on it. Face your fears, don't repress them. At the same time, as outlined in Part One, once you have sat with and faced a negative emotion, you can create a good feeling just by tuning into it.

Dealing with Birthing Fears

Whatever one is most afraid of or tense about is often the very thing that will invade one's birthing space and prevent it from going as one wishes. Even if it doesn't happen, the fear of it will cause a difficult birth. So do the inner work and face your fears to heal them. But do not get lost in shadow work, ensure that you balance it with trust, faith, and light filling.

The biggest fear in birth is often of the birthing process and pain. This is especially true if it is your first birth or if you have had a previous "bad" birthing experience. KNOW that if you follow your intuition whilst birthing, you cannot go "wrong", yet the fear of going "wrong" is the very thing that makes it go "wrong" in the first place: fear blocks the birth hormones. So take some time to tune in and release any fears of birthing itself that you have whilst working on any other fears.

"...Current consciousness is very much one of fear and distress around birth. Most women will have met their friends and family who have actually probably had a birth with quite a lot of intervention and possibly pain and distress and after which they don't feel very satisfied. Obviously when you have a nice newborn baby as the end result, you tend to forget what you went through to get there. For women who are going to try and do something different and have an ecstatic birth, you really need to prepare, because you really need to change your mind. You need to realise that most people you come across will expect birth to be painful and unpleasant..."
Valerie J Taylor, Midwife.

Remember that if you birth from a place of "I don't want this" or "I don't want that" then this will flow unproductively through the body-mind connection.

How you feel during this birth will be reflected by the birth itself: If you feel angry you will have an angry birth, if you feel cross you will have a cross birth, if you feel turned on you will have a sensual and passionate birth, if you feel afraid you will have a tense birth, and so on. If the aim is to be at peace and happy so that you have a peaceful and happy birth, you need to take the steps to shift your internal states of being from the state you want to release to the state you want to be in.

Pregnancy is the time in your life when you are **most open** to healing, so make the most of this by clearing up your old shadows, not only to create a good birth but for your own self healing. In his book "The Power of Now", Eckhart Tolle describes the shadows and fears as "ego". He believes that the female has a gift of menses and pregnancy: these are times that we are most in tune with our internal emotional states and therefore women are one step closer to enlightenment than men. Women have a monthly gift to connect and tune in to heal internal pain and shadows, which in turn makes us natural healers.

Claire was working towards having a home birth. When her waters broke she had a night of easy and lovely surges in her birthing pool. After a few hours the midwives were called and they came to examine her. She described this as being very invasive and when her surges paused as they do for all women in between stages, she went into a panic that prolonged the natural pause.

She describes it as "*I remember thinking defensively "Well, I will not have them here with you present, will I?!" The Midwives gave me 12 hours to birth otherwise they wanted induction due to risk of infection. Under extreme pressure to birth, I found that it was just not happening for me. I tried everything: homeopathy, acupuncture, I went for walks and tried giving myself healing, constantly trying to tune in, but it was not working. Eventually I just gave in to their requests and started induction, which, after a chain of horrific and painful events, ended in c-section".*

Claire stopped birthing when she was in a healthy and natural pause that she could have dropped into to, due to fear, pressure and a sense of invasion which was created by the midwife who came in to 'help'. The risk of infection is only slight, but the intervention instantly evoked fear and pressure. This story is interesting because Claire remembered a dream in which her baby had wanted to get out of her body just above her pubic bone and she was telling it not to leave that way but to go down. Maybe it was the baby's karma to birth in that way. Maybe it was meant to be part of Claire's life journey for reasons unknown. There is also the possibility that Claire's body was letting her know there was fear that needed addressing. Perhaps if Claire had recognised this issue being present in her consciousness, she could have worked with and released that fear.

In "Ina May's Guide to Childbirth", Ina May Gaskin describes an event that depicts clearly the absolute necessity for clear emotions within the birthing space, and how issues we hold can prevent relaxation and easy birth. The following woman was lucky since she was tuned in enough to acknowledge and understand the emotions and issues that were causing her pain:

"After many hours of unproductive labour, I asked her if anything was worrying her. To my surprise, she answered yes. Her mind kept going back to the wedding vows she and her husband had written for their ceremony several months earlier. She had wanted to include promises about lifetime commitment, whereas he had been reluctant to go that far. As she told me this I experienced a tingling all over my body…I consulted Stephen, my husband, who happened to be a close friend of Pamela. He offered to give the couple a chance to repeat the marriage vows that included the "as long as we both shall live" promise. When I asked them both if they were willing to do this, they agreed. Between rushes they repeated these more comprehensive vows, and within two hours their healthy son was born."

Texts such as "A Course In Miracles" teach us to dwell solely in Light, never believing in fear. If you dwell in God/Higher Self/Light, then you will have nothing to fear as no fear will be attracted to you, only God/Light/Higher Self.

Our culture is so fear-based, and we are all so conditioned by fear of pain in birth, that a 'what if?' must be cleared for all women to prepare for their sacred birth space. What if we never entertained 'what if?' but just dwelt in a place where we ALL IS WELL? Try it for a day! Try and evoke that feeling of all being well in your body, see if you can live by that feeling. Unfortunately most 'what ifs' are rooted in trauma so we have to do the inner work to target and release the root traumas, but using the 'ALL IS WELL' mantra can have power to access and resolve some inner trauma and shift the energy by inviting in gentle release and calm.

Intuition, Fear, Need and Mind Imposing

In the Ten Steps of Part One you saw the importance of tuning in, to prevent 'mind imposing' during mantra creation. It is an essential part of the emotional clearing process to fully understand the difference between Intuition, Fear, Mind Imposing and Need.

Fear - a niggling worry/something we dread.
Need - a desperate desire for something to happen, a feeling of something we can't do without.
Mind Imposing - using your mind to force/make an idea come to fruition based on need, even if it is against nature.
Intuition - a knowing that is usually without emotion, it is clear and shines and leads to the greatest good always.

Let's say during the birth process you felt "I have to leave this room now!"
Is this a fear, need or intuition, or all at the same time?

It is intuition based on something not being right and your body removing you from it for the greatest good. It is fear as there is a worry something bad may happen in that room. If a situation like this arises, how can you be sure if it is fear or intuition? Only you know. Focus on positive feeling, tune in, follow your body, shine Light through you and if you have to leave you must, otherwise you are just imposing 'all is well' when you feel it is not. You must FEEL that all is well to birth well.

Fear can be healthy. Fear is a negative emotion telling us something is wrong and we need to remove ourselves from it. Listen to fear so you can resolve it. Leave the room and go to a place you are happy or place something in the room and shine Light within using crystals until you feel protected. Always ask for signs. Higher Beings are all around you to help you, but you must invoke and ask. You must always ask for protection and ground yourself.

Fear is your friend as it is letting you know you are not in tune with your Higher Self right now.

Intuition is doing what you want, what is right for you. If you do what you want, follow your soul path, you won't get dis-ease, you won't be ill at ease, you won't get a horrible birth. Doing what you want is the fastest way to being at one - when you want to do something and it makes you feel good it is because you are following your soul path. Doing what you want does not mean doing stupid things - drop in to your heart and see what it truly wants. Sometimes doing what you want can be hard - there are many 'shoulds' in the way that make things murky. You may really want to do a yoga retreat but when it comes down to it you feel like you would rather just stay home. Really? Do you really want to stay home? Look out for blocks that tell you that you are doing what you want but actually are preventing you from doing what you really want! What would you feel like if you stayed at home? What would you feel like if you did the retreat?

Following your intuition feels positive as it leads to the path of your higher self, but this doesn't mean that your intuition only tells you what you want to hear i.e. something you perceive as "good". Sometimes your intuition may tell you something you don't want to know - that something is not working or that something is not right and it is not always something we want to face. You may perceive it as a 'bad' thing, but actually it may be a 'good' thing, we do not have all the information to judge. Remember the good-luck/bad-luck story in the introduction. Intuition is from a source of All Light and is a KNOWing.

If you have a hunch that something is not right you need to take note and act on this.

People can confuse intuition and fear. They may think "This is not an intuitive thing, it is simply that I am afraid" and keep on affirming the opposite in a mind-imposing, forceful way. But if you stay tuned in with yourself, you will know the difference.

In my birth I had a hunch that it was time to birth. I had spent three weeks stopping the midwives from intervening as I was 3 weeks past my due date, and then I knew I had to birth. I used mantra, herbs, castor oil and went into birth only after accepting my worst fear: accepting intervention in a hospital. Just as I was about to go and I had truly accepted that it would be ok, and to have intervention birth in a hospital would not mean "I had failed", and *I fully and genuinely accepted that as a possibility,* then I went into a natural birth at home!

I later discovered that my placenta had just started to decay at that time. Likewise, I had experienced a hunch not to have my waters broken and to avoid intervention *and after the birth I discovered that I had a major artery in the way.* This is not information that myself or a doctor could have known, and at one point the nurse was actually trying to break my waters but she could not find my cervix. Luckily I had done the work to be tuned in enough to know that this was not my truth. I was guided and a miracle happened to protect my baby and myself.

My fear of intervention was my friend, it helped me to stay alive, yet it also stopped me from birthing naturally and I had to overcome that exact fear and dwell in acceptance in order to birth. So I needed to Know without having to be afraid!

I have met people who also have known that their baby was not right and gone onto to have a' 'miscarriage'. (I put this in inverted commas as it is a problematic word, one that suggests the baby has been "mis-carried" by the mother, which is disempowering). This must not be confused with worry that the baby is not right, when the baby is healthy and well. That worry must be addressed if it is one you have so you can release it.

There have also been people who knew they had to go to hospital and for good reason with positive end result. They just knew and let go of their fear.

The biggest fear or hang up is the one we need to resolve the most.

Ellen really wanted a baby but it was not happening. She tried affirming with mantra, divining, herbal medicine, acupuncture and healing alongside IVF which kept 'failing'. The thing Ellen forgot to look at was her fear of never having children and that maybe she would not have children, and that that was ok. Finally when she faced that fear and accepted that it was okay not to have children, she became pregnant, but even if she had not, she would have up levelled into a new abundance after resolving her inner fear.

In my own birth, I needed to accept the concept of induction (a fear at the time) so that I could birth in a relaxed way. It was only once I had accepted induction, that I was in a position to manifest natural birth.

So, learning to tell the difference between intuition and fear is good practise for the birth situation. It takes practise and you need to tune in using the Tuning In Meditation to ask yourself what you are feeling. Knowing yourself like this is good practise for parenting as well as for birth.

If you get confused, for whatever reason (i.e. being in a situation of panic) you can ask for signs to appear, signs that you will be sure to recognise. You might say "*if this is meant to be happening for the highest good, then so be it, otherwise let a miracle occur to change the cause of actions for the highest good of all*". However, do not let the concept of fate enable you to disempower yourself: become a master of you destiny by being aware of your inner beliefs and thoughts.

Next time a situation arises, instead of haring off down the route of high emotion and reaction, instead try to take a few quiet moments to tune into your intuition.

If a fear keeps on arising, you need to work on releasing this before your birth, using the exercises in this book. You may find that the roots of the fear are not at all what you imagined, but rooted in something quite different.

The 'i-ching' works on the principle that we need to ride the 'vibe' of the moment. So whether we are stuck with our drawing or unhappy with the pain in our birth, we need to accept it to move it on. Be stuck! Be pain! Allow baby not sleeping! In my own birth, I had to accept and just be "overdue" for things to be allowed to shift and I had to accept that intervention and a hospital birth would be okay before I went on to birth happily at home!. So rather than mind imposing and forcing mantra, as one says one's mantras, we must then **allow.**

Trusting intuition and your gut can take guts. Get used to listening and tuning in: things that feel good in your tummy are right for you, things that don't are not. It sounds so simple but this is hard to live by when we have ideals, hopes, dreams, needs, responsibilities, guilt, resentment, expectations (of self and others), and lots of "shoulds" and traumas to target. It can get a bit foggy. Take time not to seek answers, but just to get clear by meditating on stillness and asking for signs for the inner. The inner knows all, all that the mind could never fathom.

Simple Intuition Exercises

Intuition always comes from a place of love.

It takes practise to decipher intuition from other ego-derived voices, feelings and desires. Start practising these exercises now to ensure that by your time of birth you are in tune with your all knowingness.

1. Start using your intuition regularly

Learn to tell the difference between your needs, desires and your knowingness by tuning in regularly to check that what you are doing right there and then hums and is right for you.

Ask, "*does this feel right? Does it hum? Is it light?*"

Always follow the light. Follow your knowing. Your intuition comes from your Higher Self and as such is always coming from a place of love, joy, kindness. It never judges or hurts. If it feels knotty or uncomfortable, then it is a trauma response of some kind for some reason. Always notice your subtle bodily, emotional and mental reactions to events, people and places and trust this.

If you are very sensitive, half the time what you feel MIGHT NOT EVEN BE YOURS but be the energy of the people and places that surround you that you are soaking up. So as you know yourself you will know what is yours and what is not, which is why daily sitting hand on heart hand on womb is so very important. Use the Higher Self meditations later in this book to tune in: you might like to imagine a wise being inside yourself, or you may just like to trust your gut feelings. Ask for signs. Close your eyes and focus on a question then open a book or pick an angel card purposefully for the answer.

2. Assume your intuition is right all the time

...and do nothing but trust it for one whole day. Vow to yourself, that all day today, whatever the cost, you will follow your intuition. Watch what happens and notice the effects and differences between gut feelings and ego desires.

3. Clear your emotions every morning

Use the emotional clearance chart to tune in properly.

When you wake up in the morning, tune in and feel the emotions within. Connect to any emotions that need releasing.

If you are unhappy, sad, fearful, anxious etc. then tune in and place a hand onto your heart and say loving words to yourself. Then ask yourself what this emotion is and give it a voice. Write about it from your heart, let it out and then try and let it go and drop into the space beyond that emotion of centredness. Bring the Light into it.

Try not to repress the emotion and ignore it or bury it; and try not to be afraid of really feeling it. This way it becomes your ally. By tuning in and feeling it, you release it and will enable yourself to birth well by being in a space of centred peace and thus allowing your intuition to be heard more clearly. When you have released all your emotions you will be able to hear your intuition from a place of clarity and love.

Exercises to Release Fear

You must **choose** now not to beat yourself up with imaging fears and 'what ifs', and thoughts of lack. This is a victim consciousness.

To love yourself means to decide now to change your present and your future by refusing to entertain lack thoughts anymore. Choose positivity and use your imagination to shine Light!

Choose fullness now.

You will create your inner beliefs and assumptions for real. What do you feel? The world is your mirror.

Base all your decisions and make your entire approach to life from an expectation of healthy pregnancy and birth at all times.

Make that vow to yourself now.

Love yourself.

You are worth this promise and this decision.

It is up to you and in your hands.

Emotional Clearance Exercise

Ten Steps to Feeling Clear
This is a version of the 10 step plan in Part One

Step One
What is wrong?
Look at your inner tensions and be honest:
I feel angry with my man for ....
I feel pain when the surges come...

Step Two
Ask for help, you can go to your safe space to do this as outlined in the exercise below:
Please, Universe, help me to resolve this situation and bring me healing and show me what I need to know to release this trauma.
My question is why do i have this pain and why cannot I not love myself more? and why do i feel this fear around pain in birth?
Please, Angels, help me to resolve this situation. I want to feel comfortable and at ease and to enjoy these surges.

Step Three
Feel it and be with it whilst breathing deeply. Breathe out the pain and breathe in the light:
I feel really, really angry and it seems to be in my tummy area. It feels big and sad. I breathe it out. I can feel dada shouting at me for being wrong and then later that happened with Mr George at school. It comes in as clammy feeling with a weird kind of stone

in it. I take the stone and bring light into it and it starts to transform slowly into a violet crystal, as it does I see dad more peaceful and i see why he did that and i can forgive him, and i see why mr george was like that and i feel more acceptance, i feel less clammy, the violet comes into the clammy feeling and shifts it, it starts to soothe and open and expand. I breathe in this violet expansion I feel so much freer.

Step Four

Where do I feel it in my body. Keep breathing it out. Give it a voice, go deeper:

I feel it in my tummy. this is where the violet is expanding, and If I give it a voice it says "how dare you, you hurt me when you separated from me" and now i see a new situation about dada when I was 2 but the violet keeps coming and this time it brings a sunflower. I feel drawn to work with sunflowers in some way. they yellow feels empowering. as i bring in the essence of sunflower I feel I can communicate calmly and clearly to my man why and how I feel upset.

It is now in my womb area and feels like a sharp stabbing pain and now I realise that was because of this tummy and clamminess. I sound it out loud and it is deep and resonating. It seems to say "it hurts to birth, it hurts to birth! I feel pressured to birth, I feel pressured to birth!" I keep breathing it out and brining in the sunflower and the violet light.

Step Five

Keep going, using more visualisation to focus on light by experiencing and focusing on your own divinity. You can literally tune in and send White Light down through your body and shine it on any fears or shadows, and even imagine placing healing crystals there - a white quartz to connect and heal with the Earth's Crystal Grid and a Rose Quartz for healing with the Divine Mother's love. Use these stones in your birth as well as imagining them whilst you are pregnant or birthing:

I am now feeling and seeing a beautiful green crystal of love being placed inside my tummy soaking up and healing all the pain with radiant light. Whenever I feel this pain, I imagine this crystal and it seems to transform it. i can now feel expansive and peaceful and no longer afraid of any birth pain and more relaxed about that

Step Six

Use acceptance and forgiveness:

I can now forgive you Dada, and Mr George too... I forgive you, and I recognise and thank you for you are all mirroring this internal state back to me and so now even though i know what you did was not okay i let you go and call my power back to me. i see it as strands of light coming back into me.

I can now thank my body for feeling this and letting me know something is amiss. I can now trust and surrender to God in the birth space, I now trust my body much more now

Step Seven
What is the opposite state of this feeling in an "I am ..." sentence?

Feeling more love for dada now as I can forgive, and now I can also be more detached and able to let him go, not wanting approval from him anymore, no longer seeking something from him that he cannot give because he does not know how. feeling love towards my self and my 6 year old self, loving and honouring myself. I am supported and loved.

Feeling relaxed and comfortable. "I am relaxed and comfortable, I let go and feel easy and pleasant sensations whilst the surges come". I keep repeating this as I roll my hips around.

Step Eight
Affirm the opposite state of being and apply it both for yourself and for the situation. Keep saying it until you really become it and believe it. Focus on this from now onwards, rather than what is wrong, focus now on what is right:

I affirm regularly "I am loved and deeply honoured by myself" and put this on the mirror to repeat daily. I also apply this to myself "I love and honour myself"

I keep repeating this as I roll my hips around. "I feel at ease with birthing, I feel at ease birthing". I really drop into the ease and pleasant feeling that I am trying to imagine.

Step Nine
See if the outside events start to mirror your new way of being. See God in everything. See the beauty in birth and the births around you. Focus on how wonderful birth is:

John treats me with respect in ways that surprise me and I recognise the love he has for me. I love myself and honour myself within all my relationships and the anger has dissipated.

I start to become comfortable and actually looking forward to enjoying the sensations of each birthing surge when i come to birth.

Step Ten
Gratitude. Give thanks and ask, how can I help?

Thank you Angels, for bringing me healing and well done to me for empowering myself to do this. Thank you to my body for being so amazing and showing me what was amiss and knowing how to birth! My body is amazing, I am amazing! thanks to those who mirror my self and are my teachers. the violet light and green crystal help me immensely and I am working with sunflowers and eating the seeds and have bought a new sunflower painting. When i look at it, it reminds me of my expansive power, its hard to explain, it just gives me that feeling of expansion in how i commune within myself

Trust and see the Light!

Journal Exercises for Fear Release

You will need your journal for the following exercises. You could record the visualisations yourself by speaking them into you phone, and then play them back. Or get your beloved to read them to you in a very slow, gentle manner.

Visualisation Journey for Birth Ease & Flow with Spirit Guides

Close your eyes and take some deep breaths.
Really take your time to sink down and relax and let go.
Imagine some beautiful stairs in front of you that you are going to climb down. The stairs are soft and warm and as you go down each step you become more and more relaxed. Count down from ten to one and when you step off the last one, you find a door. This is the door to your safe space. Open the door then close it behind you and find yourself in the most beautiful garden. This is your garden and it is a physically protected space. No one else can ever enter this garden no matter how hard they try. It is only a place of light and love, of warmth and happiness. There is no fear here because it cannot enter. This is your safe space.
You can take some time to create it if you want. Imagine what it looks like and what it contains– big or small, in nature or inside –trees, water, mountains, cushions, animals present (what?), skyline, flowers (what?) and so on. It might change as you keep returning to it.
Within this garden you will find a reclining chair in a powerful spot. This is your special chair. It is your place for recuperation, angelic healing, for vision, communion, and your seat of power. You can lie back or sit up. It may be soft or made of gold. It may fly or travel or always be contained within this garden. It is yours and it is private and it is protected because it is your seat in the heavens and can never seat another as that is against the laws of spirit. Therefore, whatever happens, you always have this safe healing space to be in.

Sit down in your special seat in your safe garden. Feel the light and the love from the seat enter your body and heal you immediately. You may see this as colour or as white light.

If you are having a healing, you may imagine tension and fear draining away and being taken away by specific beings of light and replaced with white light. You may see beings of light enter the space to help and serve and heal you. If you want, you can ask them to place their hands onto you and to give you a healing. If any beings enter your private space they do so only at your invitation and only beings of love and light may pass through the cosmic field that surrounds a sacred safe space. You may affirm and imagine this if you want.

Breathe in the warmth and the glow.

Ask for messages, in the form of images or words. These may come as answers to specific questions.

At this point you could also ask to see your inner child or to meet your inner man or woman for messages and to see what they look like or how they interact.

Ask to meet your Higher Divine Self now. Connect with your Higher I AM self, this is your divinity and god-being inside and this is your true inner wisdom.

Really connect with your I AM and just be with your self, tuning in and feeling the wisdom needed. You may picture your I AM as a wise old lady or a young queen. Or simply as a light within.

Now you can ask to meet your personal angelic birthing guide who has been specially designated to you and your baby by the angelic realms of love and light to watch over your pregnancy and birth.

Wait for messages and imagine what he/she may look like: they may be male, female, small, big, an orb or a grid. Take your time being with them. There may even be more than one being there and some of your baby's angelic guides of love and light may be present – as they are there for you both.

Now it is time for you to ask for birth holding and alignment for birth flow.

Imagine they are placing white lights and covers over you. See gold and white pouring over you like water and holding you warm like a cloak.

Spend time building up a bubble of light, cloak of light, or imagining light grid aligning you into flow – whatever it might be or whatever colour, really take your time building it and putting it in place until it is absolutely perfect and feels very aligned.

Place it around and through yourself and your baby and loved ones.

Then place it around your birth space and pregnancy.

Some people imagine a white Light spiralling up from their feet, going around their bodies seven times and then entering the head and going down through the body, deep into the ground. Imagine roots from your feet going deep in to the centre of the Earth. See yourself and your birth and your birth space deeply protected and safe. Now that you have invoked this, it will always be so.

You can easily return to this space whenever you want just by closing your eyes and asking for the cloak or imagining that you are in this space again. Just see yourself in the circle of light. You can do this in your birth or whenever you are afraid or worried about something. You can also put the light around events past and future, your children and other people, or even your car.

Give thanks and return when ready, through the door, closing it behind you, back up the stairs, and to the room you sit in. Notice things around you and breathe roots deep down into the earth. Feel the Light flow now in place around you and keep it with you for today, and always.

If you decide to have a scan, you can do this Light flow visualisation before and whilst it is happening, and tell your baby what is going on.

To align yourself very quickly you could just invoke and imagine this light flow energy by saying something three times, for example:
I call upon my Divine Higher Self and spirit guides to protect me now with love and light. I thank you and trust that it is so.

Visualisation for Fear Release

From a deep meditative place, return to your safe space by following the protection exercise above.

When you are in your chair, ask for angelic beings for release to come forward. Imagine beautiful angels coming specifically to remove any issues or tensions that you may have. You can write them down on paper or just hold them in your mind. Then give each one to your angel in your mind's eye and imagine her/him/them removing the specific fear. Ask that they may do this for the highest good of all concerned. They might take the paper in their hands or put it into a special bag. Name each fear as you give it to them clearly. Ask them that it be destroyed forever and for all good and for the opposing positive quality to arise in its place. Name what that is. Go through each fear like this. Once your angel has all the fears and you are filled with all the love and warmth, then see the angel vanish with your fears into the eternal light of "God" where they instantly vanish as they are engulfed by the light.

If you want to deepen this you may imagine such things as your fears being placed into a fire pit and a metal door shutting, after they are burnt, a wind comes and blows the ashes, breaking them up and disintegrating them into nothing.

Or you may invent your own way of imagining them going.

Just remember that once you have done this, it is done forever and you have no need to return to that fear as it has been dealt with and it is now in the past.

Give thanks.

Spend some time feeling the light and the beautiful quality that you are now filled with in place of your fear.

Be with this beautiful quality for some time.

You may ask for some sort of gift or necklace of protection to wear around you or hold, either in your mind's eye or to come to you physically in the next few days. For example, gold is an angel colour that is very protective and can keep you safe in angelic presence. Or a clear and warm crystal might come to you, such as rose quartz.

Then slowly return the way you came, shutting the door, climbing the stairs and giving thanks.

Ask for protection and ground yourself by noticing things in the room and imagining roots from your feet into the earth.

Finally notice the new quality and lightness in your being and carry it with you alongside your imaginary (or real if you get one physically) protective gift.

This situation has already been healed right now. Your fear has been released and your birth is now safe, clear and at ease. All is well for the highest good of all concerned!

So be it and so it is!

Relaxation and Love Visualisation

Now that you have released your fears, return to your garden and rest on your chair to relax deeply.

Imagine bird song, sounds of nature, a distant waterfall, feel the sun shining upon you...

Just close your eyes now and think of all the love and beauty you have ever felt. Feel it. Watch the warmth reach out towards you and take over every vibe inside every cell...it's reaching and glowing, open your arms out towards it. Just think of all that love and you will reach it. This love revolves around the planet...close your eyes, there it goes, envelop it and you will become it, floating free, high in truth. Don't let judgemental thoughts or any other thoughts annoy you. Let them float by silently...did you see it? Can you feel the love? Think of people you love, really tune into your love for them then extend that to others, to the country, to the continent, to the planet...true beauty of the land of togetherness...
Drift into lands where you tingle with love, with happiness, with dreams. Float and fly, free as you can be.
Enjoy.
Delve into the warm lap of the gods as deep as you dare.
Float and love.
When you are ready, return with the love in your heart and your belly.

Exercise in Oneness

THERE IS NO "US" AND "THEM", JUST "US".
Your mantra for the day is "You are Me and I Love YOU".
Try practising this concept for a whole day. Or try and put it into practise with your worst "enemy" – the person who triggers you the most or who you deem as most toxic. This is not to allow abuse to happen, this is to allow yourself to come out of victimhood, to see how and where you might allow any trauma and how you can have clear healthy boundaries in self love to manifest something else. Forgiveness is not saying 'that was okay' but it is saying to yourself 'that was not okay but now i can move on and it is okay that is was not okay'. There is an idea that a co-dependant and a narcissist are 2 sides of one same coin, so this is a step with the intention to come away for that coin completely, by owning our own stuff and this brings us back to our own power.

Karma Yoga
"You must be the change you want to see in the world"
Mahatma Gandhi

To see everything as a gift from God, we look for light and gifts in everything.

We have discussed Japa (repetition of mantra throughout the day). Japa is a part of Karma Yoga. Karma Yoga is about making your everyday life your spiritual practise and meditation. Like Yogi Bhajan and many other spiritual masters, Babaji came to Earth to give the massage that Karma Yoga with Japa is the only way to freedom: it is the yoga of the householder, bringing the spiritual into the every day shopping wood fetching water.

'THE POWER OF THE WORD' IS KEY IN THE AQUARIAN AGE. From now on, try practising karma yoga - make everything you do, from washing up to shopping, your spiritual practise. Spirituality does not have to be in a cave on a mountain or in a yoga room, or just in front of your birth table, it is also when you are in the office, on the phone to customer services, in the supermarket or on the train. This way you clear your karma. Bless everyone who you come into contact with, either on the phone, in a queue or passing in a car. Chant the name of Goddess as you do your chores. Turn your every day actions into spiritual practise.

Brother Lawrence, a seventeenth century Carmelite assigned to kitchen work, called this "practising the presence of God". Live your truth in everyday life, not just in your private thoughts at home. Spending your pregnancy practising all your living interactions, including parenting children as karma yoga, will set you up for a Sacred Birth. Making the profane sacred means that everything we do becomes a form of worship. Your children are your yoga.

Here is a reminder of two truths to focus upon when out in the everyday world:

> 1.   Remember to be living beyond thought, or being thought aware in all your life interactions. Think what you want to have in your life and create it with your thoughts. Then go beyond that into no thought, just being.

> 2.   Remember the message of Oneness. See God in others. The greeting "Namaste" in India means "I salute the God within You". We are all one. When you see other people's pain or "stuff", then look beyond it to the God-like selves within them. Separateness is the predominant structure in our culture of scientific materialism. Even something like astrology can stop us from being in oneness – *everything* that supports a separate identity keeps us in a separate consciousness. We are all part of the same "thing", it is our ego and our shadows that separate us.

If you met an enlightened being or God, how would you want him/her to look at you? To see how you are but to forgive you and love you for it? To talk to the real you, but be loved and forgiven for your faults? When you see faults in others, try to look beyond them and see the 'should' beneath, and also recognise that they are simply mirrors for your own ego. Yogi Bhajan only saw Lights of different colours when he spoke to people, he did not personalities.

Blessing - The Ultimate Positive Thinking for Transformation

The secret to success is to bless everyone and everything that represents what you want. To bless something is to enhance its positive quality with the intent that what is recognised will increase. This is effective, he says, because "it stirs up the positive force of the power of the universe ... and moves your energy outward". He says that you increase the same good in your own life "when you bless for benefit of others instead of directly for yourself, you tend to bypass subconscious fears about what you want for yourself".

The first step to blessing is to use the four verbal blessings:
Admiration – *what a beautiful pregnant body she has.*
Affirmation – *blessed be the ease of my birth.*
Appreciation – *pregnancy is a gift.*
Anticipation – *I wish you a beautiful baby.*

Through doing this you erase any negativity:
Admiring, instead of criticising
Affirming, instead of doubting
Appreciating, instead of blaming
Anticipating with trust instead of worrying

Since everything is one and everything is linked in the great Divine Plan, you might want to bless other things aside from birth, to further enhance your birth: health, happiness, prosperity, success, confidence, love and friendship, inner peace and spiritual growth.

Exercise for Blessing

Create some meditation space and take some deep breaths. Really relax into them.
Now begin to shine light around you. Bring it down and around you and really fill yourself up with this beautiful light.

When you feel complete and radiantly full, place one hand on the crown of your head and the other on your naval, and send the light to everyone who you would like to bless who is associated with childbirth and pregnancy in some way for you: they may be pregnant, have been pregnant, have had a baby, have children, or want to have children, as well as babies that you know…

See those beings healed and happy, surrounded by this beautiful light.

When you have done this, send light to all the happy and sad events around childbirth and pregnancy that you would like to bless, including: different types of births, images you have seen in the media related to birth and pregnancy, births that you have heard about, your own birth, your mother's birth, past births you have had yourself (or terminations and losses), menstrual cycles that you or others have experienced, other people's terminations and losses, magical births that have inspired you… See those events healed and happy, surrounded by this beautiful light.

Give thanks, and know that, for the highest good of all concerned, all these people and events are now blessed! So be it and so it is! From now onwards as you walk through life you may silently bless all who cross your path, especially people who irritate you.

Benediction
There is only One Son of God
And You are He.
From Him, you receive.
To Him, you give.
When you look at yourself
may you remember.
When you look at your brother,
may you also remember.
When you look away in fear,
remember only this:
Subject and Object,
Lover and Beloved,
are not two
but one and the same.
What you give
and what you receive
are reflections
of each other.

Paul Ferrini

We are all one. So give to yourself, give, give and give some more; and love yourself, love, love and love yourself some more... and in doing so, you are able to love and give to others. An inability to love another fully or unconditionally is an inability to love yourself.

A mother and newborn baby are so completely 'one', that whatever the mother feels, the baby will simply reflect – there is no greater time than motherhood for a reflection of ourselves and for oneness. Whatever we feel, our baby does too. Once born, the baby continues to live and feed from the Mother's auric field for many years to come. Knowing this is essential for sacred birthing, bonding and parenting... but don't beat yourself up if you have negative emotions, it does not have to be amazing all the time. Your baby/child is non–judgemental.

Babies and children are also absolutely one with the world; they have no concept of separateness from others, including people beyond the mother. A two year old has no concept of liking or disliking a person, nor the future or past, they just 'are' and they respond accordingly in the moment.

It is an important preparation for sacred birth to see the oneness in all others, as well as an essential part of self-healing and discovery.

We live in a mindset of separation and fear since our sense of community has been weakened. With our choice of objects, people and lifestyles comes freedom, but it comes at the cost of judgement, displacement, isolation etc. In *Ancient Futures*, Helena Norberg-Hodge writes about a woman from Ladakh who was vibrant, young and happy but was displaced from her community in the name of development. When the author visits her later, she lives in a house with new sofas, a new television, and new heating. But she sits alone on the floor, her husband working elsewhere, her children educated elsewhere, with the television for company and the glow in her eyes dulled.

Albert Einstein wrote about the delusion of separateness:

"A human being is a part of the whole called by us 'the universe', a part limited in time and space. He experiences himself as his thoughts and feelings, as something separate from the rest – a kind of optical delusion of his consciousness. This delusion is a kind of prison for us, restricting us to our personal desires and affection for a few persons nearest to us. Our task must be to free ourselves from this prison by widening our circle of understanding and compassion to embrace all living creatures and the whole of nature in its beauty."

This means that deep down, beneath the ego, within ourselves and others lies "God", and in that God place we are all one. It is important to get beyond ego when looking at another. To connect and see the God-Light within another, whoever they might be, will only enable them to be with it too.

This is great practise in a birthing room if you have an unwanted nurse or doctor – to connect with their God place rather than judging and reacting to their ego, by remaining in the "Om" place of alignment and flow within you (refer to the Visualisation Journey for Birth Ease & Flow with Spirit Guides). You may find that by doing this, their ego may soften or they may vanish completely if needs be. If you find yourself birthing with someone around you who you do not like, refer to a mantra that will keep you centred in the light and shift the energy. Keep chanting it within silently or just keep returning back to that place where they are at source. Practising oneness in birth means that everything will happen in flow. When you align to God, you may find the person who has an energy that triggers you will likely disappear from your energy field.

God and angelic beings do not look at your ego, nor judge it, they see beyond it and see only the light within you. Like a mother looks at her beloved child, if they see your ego (or pain-body), they look upon it with compassion, acceptance, forgiveness and unconditional and compassionate love.

"When you are looking at someone else you are really looking at nothing but yourself. All form, all separateness, is just passing show. All emotion, all relationship, is just illusion. Bodies, personalities, astrological signs, souls – it's all just yourself dancing with yourself, by making believe that you are separate".
Paths to God, by Ram Dass

"I tell you one thing. If you want peace of mind, do not find fault with others. Rather see your own faults"
The Holy Mother – Sri Saradamani Devi

In the above book, Ram Dass tells a beautiful story that represents oneness beautifully. It goes as follows:

"My father said to me "I saw those records you put out. They look great. But I can't understand: why are you selling them so cheaply? You're selling six records for four and a half dollars? You could probably get fifteen for those records – well nine anyway!"
I said, "Yeah, Dad, I know, but it costs us four and a half dollars to produce them."
He asked, "How many have you sold?"
I said, "About ten thousand."
He said, "Would those same people have paid nine dollars for them?"
I said, "Yeah, they probably would have paid nine."
"You could have charged nine" he said, "and you only charged four-fifty? What are you, against capitalism or something?"
I tried to think how I could explain it to him. My father was a lawyer, so I said, "Dad, didn't you just try a case for Uncle Henry?"
He said, "Yeah."
I asked, "Was it a tough case?"
"Oh, you bet. Very tough," he said
"Did you win it?"
"Yeah," he said, "but I'll tell you, I had to spend a lot of time on that damn case. I was at the law library every night, I had to talk to the judge – a very difficult case."
I said, "Boy, I'll bet you charged him an arm and a leg for that one!"
(My father used to charge pretty hefty fees.)
My father looked at me as if I had gone crazy. He said "What! – are you out of your mind?! Of course I didn't charge him – Uncle Henry is family."
I said, "Well, Dad, that's my predicament. If you show me anyone who isn't Uncle Henry, I'll happily rip him off."
Once it's all "us", it immediately changes the way we deal with other people."

The Golden Rule

Unitarians believe in the unity of all religions and philosophical truth that leads towards unity of man with the Divine.

Jesus	whatever you would have men do to you do also to them
Confucius	do unto others what you would not they do unto you
Laotse	regard your neighbour's gain as your own gain, and regard you neighbour's loss as your own loss.
Buddha	hurt not others with that which pains yourself
Hinduism	do naught to others which if done to thee would cause thee pain
Zoroaster	that nature only is good that does not do unto another whatever is not good for its own self.
Mohammed	no one of you is a believer until he loves for his brother what he loves for himself
Judaism	what is hurtful to yourself do not to your fellow man.

Meditation for Loving Kindness

A 2,500-year-old practice of compassion
Sit in a comfortable fashion. Let your body relax and be at rest. Let it be soft and your breath be soft. Bring your attention to the area of the heart. See if you can feel your breath coming in... and out... of your heart centre. Begin to repeat the following phrases directed to yourself. You begin with yourself because without loving yourself it is almost impossible to love others.
May I be filled with loving –kindness.
May my heart open, with kindness and peace.
You deserve it, all beings do...
May I be filled with the spirit of loving –kindness. May I be peaceful.
Feel the compassion for wherever as well, for your struggles and sorrows. We all have our pain and our sorrows. May my heart open and may I touch this sorrow with compassion and loving kindness
Sense yourself as a young child. You were a little child once. You didn't or shouldn't have had to do anything to earn love. Little children are simply there to be loved. And then with your heart hold yourself as this child with great kindness. May I be peaceful and at ease
May I be happy.
Adjust the words and images so that you find the exact phrases to best open your heart of kindness. Repeat the phrases again and again, letting the feelings permeate the body. Practice this meditation for a number of weeks until the sense of loving kindness for yourself grows. When you feel ready, gradually extend the focus of your meditation to include others you care about until eventually you include all beings everywhere. You can learn to practice it anywhere, in traffic jams, washing up, waiting to pick up your child from school. As you silently practice this loving kindness meditation among people, you will immediately feel a wonderful connection with them – the power of loving kindness. It will calm your life and keep you connected to your heart.

Loving a Challenger

A challenger is someone who"pushes your buttons". Following is a quick way to cope with a challenger in your life. A challenger is a soul working for your highest purpose, to help you overcome certain issues, so feel compassion for your challengers, and use forgiveness and blessing.

OK, so you are going to meet someone who triggers you. First go somewhere private and inhale through the nose then exhale noisily through your mouth. Repeat ten times and imagine the person happy. Really visualise this. Tune into the God within you and then the God within them, the place beyond ego where we are all one. Accept them by forgiving them for who they are since they are only a result of their experiences. How they talk to you is how they talk to themselves. Perhaps they are deeply hurt. See the bright Light within them. Hold compassion in your heart and when you meet them talk to the God within them, with love for their inability to be perfect. Let go of your expectations for who you want them to be. Why do you know better? Perhaps their way of being is necessary for some divine reason. Talk to the part of them you like. Tune into the part of them you like and override the rest, do not take it on board. Keep on breathing until you are ready to go and meet them.

Send them pink love from your heart. Send them Reiki. Send them blessings. Let them walk their path knowing that it is right for them to do so: who are you to judge it right or wrong? You do not have all the information and so cannot judge. Keep focused on a ONE attitude.

All is well in the eyes of God, all is as it should be. I love and I see only love.
I am happy with myself and others in my world around me.
So be it and so it is for the highest good of all concerned.
Amen.

Forgiveness Exercises
Forgiveness is the most important step in healing yourself.

"Forgiveness is the fragrance that the violet sheds on the heal that has crushed it"
Mark Twain

If you are aware that everything that occurs outside of you is a mirror for your internal state, then you are also aware that you draw events to you for learning. With this knowledge and with an understanding of karma, it is easy to thank people for hurting us as they are simply mirroring ways in which we hurt ourselves and lessons we need to learn in this incarnation. People that hurt us or irritate us in some way are God's teachers or Zen masters in disguise, with sticks hitting us, saying "wake up to this!"

If you are not separate and we are all one, someone who hurts you is merely mirroring something within you that we need to recognise. For example, if your lesson this lifetime is to be empowered and you feel disempowered inside, you may attract people that try and over-power us or dis-empower you.

Acceptance is a big part of forgiveness. If you can accept others for who they are and not try to make them fit into your own expectations of what they should be/do, then forgiveness follows easily. If you could all forgive your parents and children and accept them for who they are right now, the world would be a very different place. Accepting other's weaknesses and faults that irritate us is a truly challenging task. If a relative is truly hurting or irritating us we need to say "OK. I can see this is happening and I accept this is happening. Now I have woken up to it, what is this mirroring within me? How can I love this person without judgement and without expectation of how/what I think they *should* be/do according to my truth and not theirs?" Accept that another person is following their own journey, and it is right for them even if not for you. It is never better or worse than our own journey since we do not have all the information. Acceptance is not saying 'that was okay', acceptance is about returning you own power to say 'that was not okay, but i can let it go now by accepting it happened and they did that or could not meet me with that".

Anyone could be a master in disguise - and challengers are the greatest teachers for our growth.

In France there is a story about a beggar who sits under an archway (in Amiens) as a man walks past and takes pity on him, wrapping him in his cloak to warm him. That man was called Martin. Martin was a harsh roman soldier but later that night, after he had felt this compassion and helped the beggar, he had a dream in which he saw Christ wearing the very same cloak. This experience confirmed to him his devotion to all humankind, regardless of position in life. He became a saint known for his gentleness and unassuming nature, who brings light into darkness. The evening of St. Martin takes place in November when lanterns are carried into French homes in a festival of song. So the beggar has fulfilled his destiny and task for humankind – all he needed to do was to be there at that time and place for a brief instance. That was the reason for his life. All those people who judged that beggar as being a waste of time or space or a pitiful being were ignorant. This truth is important to be aware of whilst manifesting your birthing space: you go with the flow thus manifesting your positive intentions, but you also surrender to God's will for the highest good.

Everyone has a reason for doing things. If you have a problem with someone else's reason, then it is your problem, and it is one that burdens your soul not theirs. Let's not forget that "only a fool argues with a fool". You are probably also challenging this other person too, but if you deal with it and release them into light, seeing their god light and thanking them with grace, the karma will dissipate quicker and you also release them into the light. The Huna Blessing is very useful for this. Once we hold the key and understanding to forgiveness, we can release all tension, resentment and anger within our bodies and instead focus more clearly on love and gratitude. With love and gratitude we can birth easily and well since our inner rivers run clear.

If one was to take the story of Jesus the Christ as metaphor, we could see that the stage of forgiveness in spiritual development is the stage of the crucifixion. Once we can forgive our persecutors fully within ourselves then we can ascend and fly.

According to The Course in Miracles, forgiveness is the only tool to finding peace and harmony and being present. You may not even feel that you need to forgive anything or anyone before you embark on this exercise, but give it a go anyhow. Alternatively you may feel very angry towards one person but, the more you delve, find that there are other people and events, including yourself, that you blame without realising it. Resolve **all** relationships now with forgiveness. With forgiveness you will "get the past out of your present".

Forgiveness Meditation

Use the following Forgiveness Meditation alongside the Blessing Exercise in the previous chapter.

Think about what forgiveness is and what it means. Forgiving someone is different from apologising to someone. It is different from letting something that matters go. It is instead a way of connecting to the Divine and releasing/healing the karma. It is the secret for health.

Write down the name of every person who has ever hurt and bothered you. This is a big thing to do! Go through the major life events. It doesn't have to just be people, it can be events, objects and animals. You will start with a long list and the more you do the exercise, the shorter it will become. Now take this list of names and forgive each person. Hold the image of each person in your mind and affirm "I forgive you. I release any irritation or hurt that I may hold within me about you right now. Please forgive me too. I love you." Even if you do not feel you need forgiveness it is important to ask for this as by doing so you acknowledge that everything is a reflection of your inner world and therefore was created by you. We are all one! Hold the tuning-in with each name until you feel it is complete and then move on to the next.

You can do this regularly; try it before sleep each night when you reflect on your day.

Know that you are now cleansed of any resentment, guilt, anger and hurt for the highest good of all concerned.

So be it and so it is!

3 - Clear Body

"The body weeps the tears the eyes refuse to shed."
Proverb.

"I have always been bemused by the fact that many pregnant women spend longer preparing the nursery for their baby than their bodies."
Gowri Motha, *The Gentle Birth Method*

Self Nourishing Tools

Learn about the changes that take place in your pregnant body and about your baby's growth patterns. The more you know about your body in birth, the more empowered you can be when making decisions and creating personal visualisations.

After twenty eight weeks of pregnancy, you and your baby have reached a landmark and your baby is now getting ready for life on the outside of the womb. Their lungs have now started to secrete a protein that helps them to take their first breath. Now is the time for focusing on creating more space for your baby to grow to the maximum and perfect size.

Imagine all the positive growth events and changes that are occurring in your baby and love yourself too. Since a pregnant woman constantly communicates telepathically with her baby, loving yourself sends deep positively affirming signals to your baby. Now is the time to groom and love every bit of your body, to truly feel like a woman in the following ways.

Self Grooming
Groom and love your body with essential oils, baths and massage as well as wearing light, flowing beautiful clothes rather than heavy dark ones. Use crystals in the bath as well as spending time in meditation and reading good books. Have your partner massage you in the bath.

Oils to avoid in pregnancy include: aniseed, basil, camphor, caraway, cedar, cinnamon, clary sage, cypress, fennel, hyssop, juniper, marjoram, myrrh, nutmeg, oreganum, peppermint, pennyroyal, rose, rosemary, sage, savoury, thuja, thyme, wintergreen.

(However, I LOVED using rose in pregnancy – some of these recommendations are not scientifically based and it is useful to consult an aromatherapist).

Frankincense and patchouli mixed into a gentle carrier/base oil like vitamin E, almond or grape seed makes a good massage oil or pregnancy:

Crystals for pregnancy: moonstone, azurite, unakite, rose quartz.

Massage

Try out functional massage for toxin release and body stimulation, as well as intuitive and loving pregnancy massage for sending loving vibrations to both your body and your baby.

It is important to remember that during massage the words that you hear can have deep and profound effects on your body. Therefore, pick a practitioner who is aware of this and can either speak or think positive beautiful words. You can either use the time to switch off or to say your mantras or do the visualisations.

Indian Head massage can really help you to feel like a beautiful woman.

Perineum massage is to be started from week 36 (not before) and outlined fully in the connection chapter since it is something you might like to share with your birth partner.

Daily self massage whilst talking to your baby and cervix is also talked about in the connection exercises. You can ask your cervix to open and thin from week 38. This is outlined in the meditation on healthy pregnant body.

Alternative Therapies

There are many therapies which can offer relaxation throughout pregnancy as well as being used to address specific issues which may arise. The convenience of a practitioner's location for you and your life is an essential consideration, as well as the vibe of the therapist. If it is a difficult place or time for you to get to, then it will not enable you to heal and relax but merely create tension.

You have every right to cancel any treatment if it does not feel right. Even if it is less than 24 hours' notice, do it anyway – even if you need to pay for the treatment, as it is essential you follow your intuition. If a practitioner does not understand then they are not the right person for you.

Nutrition

Nothing is right or wrong but I strongly suggest thinking about eliminating wheat and sugar, and possibly dairy. You could see a kinesiologist for testing, or else use the intuition exercises and do it yourself.

Make changes subtle at first. For example, if you were a serious meat eater with a tobacco and chocolate diet, and suddenly moved to a pure, raw-only, organic diet overnight, you might experience illness. Doing it in stages is the way forward. Keep on following the energy. Some people can live on nothing but light, because that is where they are at right now. Others could not. Some people need meat. Others need fish. Some people get to a stage where they want only raw, then need to go back to fish again…it all depends on tuning in to where your energy is right now and being aware that this might shift at any given moment.

Pregnancy is the time to eat all those healthy fruits and vegetables, and for some, meat too. Eat foods that are as alive as possible, raw or lightly steamed. Drink lots of water or herbal tea.

Try juicing vegetables and wheatgrass for optimal health. A pint glass of fresh juice a day mixed with a high quality superfood powder is the best thing you could do for your baby and body - juice carrots, apples, celery, parsley, beetroot, ginger (all organic) every morning. You can save the pulp of the veg and blend with other things (ground flax, olives, sun dried tomatoes, tomatoes, ground almonds etc.) and mix into raw burgers and dehydrate (if you don't have a dehydrator just use the oven on very low). Get a masticating juicer that enables you to juice leaves and retains the vitamins and minerals. They are an investment but a good one to make and it will keep you going while breastfeeding, chasing toddlers or getting up early for school runs…and beyond!

You can easily grow your own wheatgrass. I recommend looking at some raw food books for ideas on maximum natural vitamin supplementations, as opposed to artificial ones.

Suggestions for Superfood to Supplement your Body during Pregnancy

- Raw cacao (if you must have it, eat raw cacao instead of chocolate, you can
- get some delicious ready made raw bars)
- Maca - this is a root vegetable from peru full of vitamins, minerals and enzymes and all eight amino acids
- Algae and seaweed
- Wild foraged food
- Powered green superfood (such as spirulina or barleygrass)
- Carob powder
- Good oils - flaxseed or hemp oil
- Seeds - hemp seeds, linseeds. My friend believes that her wrinkles physically diminish after eating hemp seeds!
- Buckwheat - you can soak the seeds and the buckwheat overnight and eat raw the next day
- Nuts and nut butters - I ate them, but trust your feelings
- Himalayan pink salt - instead of refined salt
- Sprouts
- Ho shou wu - a Chinese youth giving tonic
- Agave nectar, honey, molasses, maple syrup - instead of sugar
- Bee pollen
- Lucuma powder
- Raw vegan pesto
- Mesquite meal - high protein and mineral content
- Ginseng
- Berries - blueberries, acai and goji berries
- Purplecorn
- Salba / Chia seeds
- Digestive enzymes - sprinkle on food;
- Etheriums / Colloidal silver, a heal-all

Iron and zinc rich foods are essential for the growing baby. Find iron in eggs, molasses, dried fruits, leafy vegetables, beans and lentils. Zinc is in almonds, avocado, cheese, lentils, bananas, sesame seeds, sunflower seeds and haricot beans. From 28 weeks your baby needs extra calcium: fish, dairy, watercress, oats, millet, green leafy vegetables. Avoid coffee, which prevents absorption of nutrients, and fizzy drinks, which actually deplete calcium from your body.

From 28 weeks, you could follow a yogic diet.

The Yogic Three Guanas - Sattvic, Rajasic and Tamasic

Sattvic food is the purest diet and calms the mind and body, enabling you to function to maximum potential with true health so that pure energy can flow between mother and baby. This includes organic and locally or well sourced fresh cereals, bread, fruit, vegetables, milk, butter, cheese, legumes, nuts, seeds, honey, some herb teas and superfoods such as those mentioned above, focusing on eating with stillness and presence.

Rajasic food is hot, bitter, sour, dry or salty and destroys the mind-body equilibrium, over-exciting and over–stimulating, causing restless minds. These foods include hot and sharp spices and herbs, stimulants like coffee, tea, chocolate, eggs, fish and salt and this is compounded by eating in a hurry, talking too much or reading (not being present with your food).

Tamasic diets benefit neither mind nor body, and create inertia and disease by withdrawing "prana" (or energy) and clouding the mind with dark emotions. These include meat, tobacco, alcohol, onions, garlic, fermented foods, overripe, overcooked, over manufactured or processed food and food grown with chemicals or genetically modified ingredients. This is characterised by over eating.

I suggest following gentle, easy programmes that make you feel at ease and happy, rather than extreme nutritional diets and exercise regimes that you feel under pressure to stick to.

Follow your intuition since something that is good for one body is not always right for another. Many healthy body books generalise about the human body. However, we are all different and all have differing needs. Of course, some things are obviously poisonous or harmful for all pregnant women (possibly the harmful herbs listed below) but other things can't be generalised about: every individual has differing life experience, body make up, genetic imprints, levels of emotional support, geographical conditions, family and life circumstances etc. Therefore, follow your intuition and gut instincts about what is right and wrong for you in every circumstance, be it a yoga class, nutritional regime or in the birthing space whilst talking to a doctor. Follow guides but ensure that you personalise them.

For example, you may feel that a strict non-sugar diet is absolutely necessary for you, and in following it you may even uncover certain issues that led you to binge previously. Or you may feel the necessity to eat and enjoy whatever you like: just be honest with yourself. You know if it is good for you or not deep down. You know if it is ok to treat yourself and when to do it. You Know.

It is mostly about balance: being healthy, yet letting go and not being too rigid about things. Also notice your attachment to certain foods: if you are attached to something, you may find that you need to learn to let go of that very thing. A craving often indicates a deficiency or an imbalance - a craving for sugar often comes with candida since the candida needs the sugar to feed on. . Alternatively you may find that an ingredient within your food is the thing you are craving and that you can happily replace it with something else. Just be loose though! Pregnancy preparations are about clearing our channels, but also about being happy and loving ourselves. Try and fill up from the inside rather than looking to consume substances in order to fulfil an inner need.

You could try approaching certain things you do with "If I loved myself I would…." This can help you with certain nutritional decisions alongside kinesiology or a visit to a nutritionist.

If you are craving a certain food like chocolate, you could meditate on why this is. Do the tuning-in meditation and ask questions such as: Do I need the magnesium it contains? Is it ok for me to eat it regularly? Some people believe that chocolate represents a need for love and romance. What does it mean for me?

I have found through personal experience that when I crave something it is because I believe somewhere deep down that it is delicious and a treat. One can crave things from an inner energetic trauma making one believe they want it. However pregnant women often crave things not based on false desire and trauma but on actual bodily needs, so you have to tune in to understand what is the root cause of the craving.

For example, I was conditioned to believe that a chocolate brownie was a special treat, a 'pick me up', that it is absolutely yummy. So I bought one to fill a need in me that is actually about wanting love – I need filling up quickly in some way with something that makes me feel good. The same happened with a previous tobacco habit. If I tried to give up these treats, not only was I preventing myself from something special and yummy (like love and inspiration, which I really needed) but I was "giving up" or "starving" myself of something which I believed to be good. I was not targeting the inner trauma and until I did that I would replace one habit or craving with another.

When I finally targeted my inner emotional trauma, I was able to "easily let go" instead of "give up". It was easy since not only did I have the will to do it (I genuinely wanted to for myself because it did not feel right inside my body any more) but I now believed that it was not enjoyable. Chocolate went from something yummy to something disgusting: the bitter, fat, sugar all tasted like toxins and actually made me feel repulsed! And tobacco…Yuck!

However until I healed the inner trauma, I replaced the 'unhealthy' habit with 'healthy' eating and drinking lots of fresh spring water, but found that the obsession for chocolate and tobacco was replaced with an obsession for organic-only local food since I believed that this was the only thing that was now a treat. This was not very healthy either as I was still filling up from the outside. I was replacing one need with another need rather than filling up from within.

We can only balance the extremes when we target the trauma.

I am using chocolate as an example, some pregnant women need chocolate for the magnesium or pick me up and it can be a genuine desire rather than a trauma desire. So you have to know your own gut and be honest with yourself.

Everything that believe stems from inner root core emotions, and this affects **everything.**

If you have a craving you wish to target and heal, resolve it now by using the Ten Step Birthing Mantra Creation Plan to understand, heal and change your core root feelings and beliefs around it.

Finally, remember that a good diet is also one that eats blessed food with Love. Be aware of your mental and emotional states as you eat your food and of the emotional states which your food may be feeding.

Herbs and Homeopathy

Find a specialist or a good book and tune into your instincts. If you see a homeopath, s/he will go into your entire history to find the right remedy especially for you, therefore I do not list general ones for pregnancy related ailments here.

Some herbs, and almost all medication, are **not recommended** in pregnancy for ALL people. The herbs to avoid are as follows: aloes, barberry, black cohosh, bloodroot, buckthorn, cascara sagrada, cinchona, cottonroot, golden seal, greater celandine, juniper, liferoot, male fern, mandrake, pennyroyal, poke root, rhubarb, rue, saffron, sage, southernwood, tansy, thuja, wormwood.

Others are debated, for example you can purchase a herbal tea formula for womb preparation that includes raspberry leaf from week 12, whereas some people say raspberry leaf should not be taken until the third trimester. You can also buy ayurvedic formulas and tissue salts that have been specially prepared for the pregnant body and growing baby, as well as ayurvedic oil that can be used to massage the perenium from week thirty six.

Physical Exercise

Keep it gentle but take it every day – a rough guide for this stage in pregnancy could be a brisk walk of thirty minutes a day, twenty minutes a day of yoga, swimming once weekly if you can find a pool that is relaxing and not too chlorinated. There are simple exercises outlined in most pregnancy books if you want to follow a daily routine.

Do pelvic floor muscles every time you make tea or whenever you think of them: squeeze your anal, vaginal and urinal passages at separate times. Use emptying your bowels as an exercise in relaxing and visualising things coming out smoothly, rather than pushing and straining. The perfect chance to practise for birth!

Pregnancy Yoga

Start a class now if you have not already. There will be a class near you. Try out several since they all differ.

You may or may not want to mix with the other pregnant mothers and that is fine, but it is lovely to be in a room in silence with lots of other birthing women and strength can really be drawn from that experience alone. The exercises will also prepare and keep your body supple and nurtured ready for birth.

A good practitioner will be ready to support and help with holistic birth enquiries. There will also be notice boards advertising therapists who work with pregnant women in your area.

Make sure you follow your body and never do anything that does not feel right, whatever the yoga practitioner says. Only you know your body, your life and your baby.

Surrendering to your Body

You must surrender to your body and learn to trust it. In birth, your body knows exactly what to do. As preparation for birth and for a healthy pregnant body, close your eyes go on all fours and start to move as your body wants you to and as you do so, affirm *"I turn birthing over to my body. My body knows what to do"*

Ina May Gaskin writes: *"Let your monkey do it. Letting the primate in you do the work of labour is a short way of saying not to let your over-busy mind interfere with the ancient wisdom of your body. To give you an idea of what I mean, here are some things monkeys and apes don't do that many women do – and that interfere with labour:*

Monkeys don't think of technology as necessary to giving birth
Monkeys don't obsess about their bodies being inadequate
Monkeys don't blame their condition on anyone else
Monkeys don't do math about their dilation to speculate how long labour might take (…)
Monkeys in labour get into the position that feels best, not the one they're told to assume.
Monkeys aren't self conscious about making noise, farting, or pooping during labour…"

Ina May Gaskin, *Ina May's Guide to Childbirth*

Exercise for Body Surrender

Get onto all fours and close your eyes.
Take ten deep breaths and tune into your Hara (below your tummy button). This is your centre.

Start to move from there, slowly in tune with the breathing. You may want to circle your hips in very small circles, move fast or slow, move your legs. Keep on breathing from your Hara. You may want to shake some tension out with short fast breaths and kicks of the legs, or roll around the floor.

Surrender to your body, let it take over. Become a wild animal, a monkey. Override your busy mind and let your body do what it wants to do without judging it in any way.

You may want to say some healthy body affirmations at the same time, either personal ones for health, or general ones such as "I turn birthing over to my body, I surrender easily to my body, I love my body, my body knows". Or chant "Ram!" or "I love my beautiful glowing body!"

You could also go into more specific body parts such as "I love my beautiful face, thank you beautiful face!" and so on. I love my beautiful neck, thank you beautiful neck! I love my beautiful colon, thank you beautiful colon! I love my beautiful heart, thank you beautiful heart! I love my beautiful liver, thank you beautiful liver!"

Keep your eyes closed for the entire time while you do this exercise. This will help you tune in and is also a good trust exercise for your body. Your body knows what is around you better than your mind.

Do this for as long as you feel able to and keep coming back to this exercise regularly.

When you feel ready to finish, lie on your back or return to all fours and give thanks to your beautiful, healthy body and your healthy, beautiful baby.

Congratulate your body for doing so well and marvel at it for knowing what to do. It is growing a baby. It has been menstruating in preparation for this for many years! Your body is amazing! Thank your body and let it know that you totally trust and love it and that you will surrender to it in the birthing space.

Finally, listen to see if your body has any messages for you, or anything it wants you to do for it.

Your body can now surrender in the birth for the highest good of all concerned! So be it and so it is!

Body Healing

Remember that anything that needs healing in your body is about HOW YOU FEEL in your mind, emotions and spirit.

Anything that needs healing is called dis-ease because it is not at ease for some reason. Once the emotional ease in that place returns, the illness vanishes.

You may choose to focus on the healing of the body with herbs, medicine, nutritional advice, or a practise such as Alexander Technique; or to focus on the mind with affirmation and mantra; or the emotions with meditation and relaxation; or the spirit with Reiki and Energy Healing. Whatever you feel drawn to do - whether you approach your healing from the level of the body or/and the level of the spirit, be sure you focus on HOW YOU FEEL.

When seeking to understand illness, it can be useful to look at the PURPOSE of the dis-ease as opposed to the REASON.

If anything in the outside world that happens to us is a mirror for our internal emotional state, and vice versa, then you can apply your mantra creations to understand, heal and love your body, as well as to create a happy birth.

Applying the Mirror Concept for Treating Dis-ease

As within so without

Remember this mirror concept that your body is a mirror for your emotions and your mind. If you were constantly digesting ideas about things, then this may manifest in the body as digestive issues. If you are constantly digesting issues about protecting ourselves against other people, this may manifest as a bloated abdomen (protecting against invasion). This method can be applied to everything. The part of the body that is affected is directly connected and representational of the emotion, and vice versa.

Some examples might be:

Legs	moving / walking
Boils	anger
Back	support
Reproductive issues	gender and sexuality issues
Female problems	rejecting the feminine

Tune into yourself in meditation, to find the necessary mantra for release and healing. Then look up the herbs and homeopathic remedies that could also support your releasing work.

You are looking to shift the way of being. For example, if you have headaches, you need to shift the migraine personality into a peaceful way of being. This means noting down and altering your inner mental chatter.

Constantly imagine your body healthy and vibrant. Comb through it with your mind's eye, and see it full of white light. If you find an area that has a shadow, work through that shadow by asking what the message for you may be, using the ways we have already discussed in the Emotional Clearance Chart.

I am so happy to be able to share Jill's story with you here, because Jill followed the techniques in this book to clear a blocked fallopian tube. When going for IVF, Jill was informed that she had a blocked fallopian tube. She associated this with blocked creativity and started to affirm that she was in the flow creatively. She also saw the links between blocked creativity and her need for a baby that was not happening. She affirmed how creative she was, as well as tuning into her needs for a baby and finding the right mantras for this. As she dived into meditating with this, she then found core trauma beliefs in an old emotional feeling that she contacted and felt into and brought the light into it daily for a week. She also had energy healing session several times to tackle the root feeling with some support, and took some herbs that were relevant. She constantly imagined her tubes clear and flowing daily whilst taking up creative hobbies and classes. Then she noticed some "discharge" in the toilet with some sort of tissue in it. The following week she went for the operation to clear the tubes and they could not find anything: her tubes were no longer blocked!

Ten Steps to Self Healing with Visualisation

Use the following visualisation to heal your physical body alongside the internal work of clearing emotions and thoughts.

1. Have a hot bath and massage the area that hurts or that needs it most. Go into a deeply relaxed space using your breath and protect yourself.

2. Tune into the parts of your body that are upset. Have a conversation with them. Ask why they are unhappy; ask whether memory or thoughts that you carry have created this. Ask for the purpose rather than the reason. Ask for a good mantra to come to you. Listen carefully to any feelings that arise or words that you hear about the area and the mindset/ energy behind the discomfort.

*3. Affirm positive words and mantras that are appropriate **whilst massaging the area**. Refer to Part One.*

4. Ask for light flow and imagine light flowing around you, aligning you.

5. Ask for the help of your spirit guides and anyone else you would like to come and help and guide you through visualisation. For example, Imagine you cut open the area and take out the discomfort. The darkness that is removed could be in the form of a snake or sticky mass… whatever comes to mind and go with it. Keep pulling it out and give it to one of God's helpers and your guides to take away. This may be an angelic being or a dragon, whatever comes to mind, however crazy it might seem. See this being put the darkness into a bucket and take it away to the light to be transformed into light or zapped by a flame of Light into nothing.

6. Now fill the area up with Light. Imagine Angels and God pouring white and golden light into the area, mending and cleansing it. Now sew it up.

7. Now invoke angelic beings or more healing energy by choosing to use Reiki, Angel healing, the Violet flame (see chapter on spirit and other visualisations in this book) or just simply asking love and Light healing energy to come forward to heal you now. Archangel Raphael is the angel for healing, and your guides will clear away any residue.

8. You are now filled with Light. Be in that space. Give thanks. You are healed now and you deserve to be healed now. You are a child of God who deserves to be in the Light. Affirm, "for the highest good of all concerned the … in my …. has now gone". Refer to any illness or pain as "the…" or "a…" rather than "my…" – disown it, and keep it in the past tense if you must discuss it. So be it and so it is.

*9. Try using the words, "I am a master, and I **allow** myself to be healed." Keep in the Light, keep massaging with breath and keep any mantras and words that arise with you.*

10. When you have finished, keep visualising positive imagery. You may wish to imagine your cells glowing with Light. Keep this image and hold it in your mind constantly throughout the day as well as in meditative states, before sleep, on waking and during massage.

I am healed, so be it and so it is, Amen!

To do a quick body scan whilst out and about, just imagine White Light coming down through the top of your head, through the centre of your body and down through the ground. Wherever it gets stuck in the body, shine the Light there and place a healing crystal there in your imagination, then affirm a relevant mantra. Also refer to Quick Body Scan Drawings in Part One.

The Womb Light Visualisation

Similar to the Meditations presented in Part One, this is another visualisation to tune in and talk to your body to see what is going on, and to ensure optimum health for you and your baby, but focuses more on the womb.

Do this visualisation regularly – either over a half hour period or a five minute scan when in the bath, at traffic lights or in a yoga class; and especially whenever you look in the mirror.

Get into a comfortable position, one that you can stay in for a while.

Close your eyes and take some deep, relaxing breaths.

See any tension drain away.

Just sit with this for a while and don't rush onto the next step. This is a big part of the process.

Just keep on breathing.

You may like to go to your safe protected space: down the stairs, through the door, into your special garden and onto your chair. Ask for protection.

Now start to focus on your body. Imagine that your body is a river. See how it flows and if it runs clear. Notice the spots where the water is quiet, fast, bubbling, muddy, clear, cold, stagnant, free flowing water or water falls. Like in the tuning-in meditation, you can do a quick body scan drawing at this point.

When you have completed this, take the time to clear away any debris and to send love, Light and healing to the areas which need it most.

When you have done this, imagine that your body stands in front of you in its most radiant and healthy abundant state. See how it looks, how your belly looks, how it shines, how that feels, how your skin glows and how your muscles are toned. Really imagine your body in optimum health, right in front of you now.

Now ask that this be so now. Step inside the radiant body that stands before you… how does it feel? Become it right now as if you are putting a new skin on. You may feel the old skin shedding away or even see it peeling off and into the earth right now.

Now, imagine that a tap has been switched on above your head, sending a flowing stream into the top of your head, a flow of pure, abundant, clear and light water from the Angelic Christ realms.

See this water pouring forth, through your head and into your body.

It enters every organ, every cell, every DNA structure…

As it enters each organ, imagine it cleansing and purifying whilst simultaneously thanking each and every organ for the work that it is doing…first through your veins and into your head, eyes, hair, ends of your hair, eyelashes, pupils, ears, nose, tongue, teeth, jaw, neck, throat, shoulders, arms, elbows, hands, fingers, nails, chest, breasts, nipples (at this point imagine the abundant fantastic work that your breasts are doing in preparing for milk-supply), heart, lungs, stomach, solar plexus, abdomen, colon, intestines, kidneys, bladder, anal canal, reproductive organs (at this point see the amazing work that your body is doing in holding and growing your beautiful glowing baby within your shimmering abundant womb), sphincter muscle, perineum, vagina or yoni, pubic bone, legs, knees, ankles, feet, toes, and toe nails... not to mention all the cells, tissues and DNA structures within your body.

Now return to your reproductive organs and imagine that your womb is a beautiful cave. Go inside your womb and see this clear Christ water cleansing and purifying every corner of your womb, your baby, the placenta and the cord so that all the substances that enter your baby through the cord are purified. You could even place a filter of light there to ensure this. Really spend time inside your womb, cleansing it. If you want, you could ask a beautiful angel to come forth and stand guard at the entrance to your womb and place her wings around your womb as protection.

Imagine your baby truly glowing and growing beautifully and happily. Talk to your baby and thank her/him for coming to you. See the cord connecting you glowing with light and your placenta lovingly holding and supporting your baby. Your womb is full of Light.

Affirm a beautiful birth. You will return to this place again soon in the Baby Connection Visualisation and for your Birth Visualisation, but for now fill your baby with the beautiful water and ask for any messages to come to you.

Once you feel like you are truly glowing in every part of your body, you may return from your garden, through the door, closing it behind you, and up the stairs back to the room in which you now sit.

When you return you bring your glowing radiant body with you.
1.   Open your eyes and come back, then go to a mirror.
2.   Look at yourself and your body in the mirror and see yourself glowing.
3.   You are now full of 'womb-light'.
*4.   If you notice critical judgements of your body (my nose is wonky, my belly is too big/small for the stage I am at, I am putting on too much weight, my belly is too low, my breasts have become very big, etc.) then you need to redo the visualisation until you are feeling **100%** confidently happy with your beautiful body.*
5.   Affirm "this... is a ... of God's since I am a child of God. It is therefore beautiful and I am therefore beautiful. I love this... as I love God"
6.   You are aiming to be at optimum radiance and to be aware of it.
7.   Your nose may not be symmetrical or your belly might be hanging low, but isn't it beautiful and radiant and doesn't it glow? Really feel beautiful.
8.   Affirm to yourself as you look in the mirror: "I am radiant, my pregnant body is radiant, I glow, pregnancy becomes me, I feel energised by pregnancy, I love myself and I look after myself, I am beautiful because I am a child of God and all God's children are beautiful, like all trees big and small are beautiful, look how my beautiful body nourishes and grows a glowing radiant baby, thank you body...THANK YOU BODY!"

If you notice doubt, then deal with it, don't repress or ignore it. Wherever you go, keep the river with you and access the cleansing running water whenever you want and whenever you think of it.

You may like to have a special face cream and body oil that you fill with this water with your mind's eye. You could even place it on top of your birthing alter, above an angelic image or crystal. Every day when you put it on and lovingly rub it in, you can talk to your body and to your baby with words of gratitude and images of radiance, alongside your affirmations.

Know that you are now cleansed and radiant for the highest good of all concerned!

So be it and so it is!

Make this a part of your daily visualisation: this is something to start doing every day or more. Start massaging your belly and talking to your baby and body each day as you massage, even for just two minutes a day. While you are doing this massage and mantra you can start using the following visualisations:

1 Loosen your pelvic muscles. From twenty eight weeks you can also start to imagine your pelvic tissue and muscles becoming soft like jelly and tell them that this is so. Your body will do what you tell it to do.

2 Perfect positioning. Start to visualise your baby's position in the womb. Imagine and ask your baby to face the "right" way around. Most books, for ease of drawing and understanding, show the baby the "wrong" way around in the womb: they depict a baby so that you can see its face in the drawing whereas in fact you need to imagine your baby with its head facing towards your bottom. Imagine your baby facing the "right" way around while at the same time affirming and trusting that your baby is in the optimal birth position for a natural, easy and healthy birth.

3 Softening your cervix. From 38 weeks imagine your cervix softening and thinning now in preparation. Tell it to do so. See your cervix as golden and healthy, thinning to the right degree.

Excess Weight in Pregnancy and Breastfeeding Years

Weight and beauty is defined by culture and trend, but you know when you are healthy and when you are not. In some cultures, a large woman is considered beautiful. 'Fat' in a place where food is scarce is often associated with beauty, whereas in a culture where food is plentiful, thin is seen as more beautiful.

In my mind there is only one beautiful - when you *feel* beautiful - when you feel clear, healthy and well, regardless of weight.

Pregnant woman put on weight for various reasons which can be natural, healthy and good for mother and child. Our culture seems to see anything that is associated with extreme femininity as vulgar: large breast, large bottoms, big thighs and large post pregnant bellies. This is a result of a combination of influences including Victorian values, class values, male values and so on.

Excess oestrogen produced at this time is the cause of cellulite. If you put on weight or get excess cellulite, please don't feel anxious about it, since if you do you are denying your beautiful female self, that self which birthed your baby. When breastfeeding, you need good nutrition; it is not the time to diet. It is often exhaustion which leads to overeating (needing energy fixes) as opposed to breastfeeding, so if overeating is an issue look at how you could get more support to get more energy and more sleep.

However, have you noticed how many gurus and parents (men and women) have larger bellies? They are holding energetic space for others and often the two go hand in hand.

You are a child of God and, all children of God come in different shapes and sizes, none are better or worse and all are beautiful. Avoid media and mindsets that say one is more beautiful than another. Avoid mindsets that believe childbirth (pre and post) figures are vulgar. Allow your body to let go and do its thing. Similarly, if you do not put on weight, it is also vital to remember to honour your body for what it is and trust that your body is beautiful how it is: you are the right size for you and you are the unique you! You know if you are overeating or not. It is quite simple, you are either clearly connected within, beautiful within, or there is a block that needs addressing. If you do not feel beautiful, you need to re-connect within.

Tune in. Are you feeling healthy? Do you feel happy about just letting yourself be "new mother size" for a while? When you are "in the cave" int he first few years, perhaps you need to ground and let loose? The time will come for exercising. Or do you feel that you need to keep focused and in control of your weight? Sometimes people who shave large bellies are holding the spiritual auras of those around them, mothers can be like many spiritual masters with big bellies! Also ask yourself - are you comparing, judging or accepting yourself? Ironically you will reach your ideal weight when you love and accept who you are. Are you feeling bad about yourself - comparing yourself to ideal and unrealistic models of women that are photo shop enhanced and have possibly undergone surgery?

If you are overeating or under exercising and your weight is not healthy, you will know intuitively, and can use steps in this book to overcome any issues that may be causing this. Overeating and odd cravings in pregnancy could be the result of a mineral or vitamin deficiency or extreme exhaustion, or could be an attempt to fill up an emptiness within. Only you know. Be wary of binging whilst breastfeeding, but at the same time this is a time to be easy on yourself, and to love yourself. Sometimes when breastfeeding you can give all your love to your baby and be running on empty and the quickest way to fill up is from 'without'. If this is happening, try to notice and find other healthy ways to fill up - massage, meditation, visualisation, rest.

If you want your life to be a certain way after your pregnancy, you can use the manifestation and mantra exercises in this book but be careful you are not mind imposing due to fear. Always tune in to see if this is right for you - always use your intuition, always connect to your true beauty within! Mothers need nourishment, and this means different things to different people, we are all unique!

4 - Clear Spirit

Communicating and Connecting with Universal Spirit

Intuition derives from the place of inner stillness where we connect to the Light. Also known as God, Light, Higher Self, One Love, the all-powerful vibrations of love that connect and emanate throughout the universe, Source, Universe, Be-ingness, Christ energy, I am vibration, Divine Self and of course the Divine Mother within...

Most world religions and alternative healing therapies share the same focus: returning to the path to love, to source. All the religions of the world, all the ancient spiritual pathways, and all healing modalities around the world use different techniques and call it different names, to do this one and the same thing. We no longer need to commit to a specific religion or another person to talk to God, we can talk directly to God ourselves through meditation in any ways we so wish. It is very common for pregnant women to open to the Divine Feminine aspect of God, to align to the many Goddesses that have held birthing women through out time. This is the perfect time to be surprised and to be open to the varied forms of manifestation in which Light communes with you.

Find your inner source by connecting to anything that resonates for you during your birth. The possibilities are limitless. It may be nature, universe, trees, sunshine, Goddesses, Angels, Masters, Avatars, Mothers of Light, Beings of Light and Love, Ascended Beings, Archangels, Saints, Devas, Deities and Gurus to whom you feel most drawn to connect to. You might choose to birth as a Christian, or as a Muslim, or a Buddhist, it might surprise you in the moment, be open and whatever intuitively draws you in the moment is beautiful and perfect.

Pregnancy is THE time for you to communicate with your inner beings of Light that are there to support and love you and your baby. As you communicate, keep it light and clear and use healthy grounding. There is great power in communicating with Goddess - be clear and set the space properly with respect.

Prayer = Words of Power

If you have been practising this book's exercises in *Japa*, oneness, blessing, forgiveness and so on, you have been clearing your emotions and your spirit. If you have started saying your mantras, you will have realised directly through experience that words hold great power. Your mantras are prayer. The difference between seeing them simply as mantra and seeing them as prayer, is in perception. If you perceive that your mantras are prayer, then they will hold a greater power.

When prayers aren't answered it is because they express and affirm a lack and a need, which is then mirrored back. So take care to express a "having" attitude in your emotions, words and your prayers. It is all about positive intention. And connecting the though to the root inner subconscious belief and energy patterning within. The words must be felt, they must come from a quantum inner place. This is essential to the success of this programme and you will be returning to this quantum practise often in the exercises throughout this book.

Prayer includes the following six principles:

1. Praise and thanks.
2. Invocation of Light on Earth; invocation of Light Beings.
3. Imagining worthiness of abundance; stating specific outcome for highest good.
4. Forgiveness, acceptance and one-ness.
5. Healthy Boundary & Clear alignment & grounding (which is better than fear-based protection).
6. So be it and so it is for the highest good.

This is the same as the format in Creating Your Sacred Space - Daily Birth Preparation. So you have already been praying. This format is ancient practise seen in the ancient spiritual pathways throughout the world in varied forms and is the divine law and basis of manifestation. When the manifestation techniques become prayer they hold great power because we surrender to the Divine with trust and knowing. The key to manifestation is to go beyond words and mantras into the inner work of releasing inner blocks, old belief systems, shifting the inner energy patterning, and when we do this and combine that with the manifestation words to become a prayer, we then give it to the sacred and then it becomes all-powerful.

The 6 principles above are found in most basic prayers.

The Lord's Prayer
Our Father, who art in Heaven,
Hallowed be Thy name.
Thy Kingdom come.
Thy Will be done, on Earth as it is in Heaven.
Give us this day our daily bread.
And forgive us our trespasses,
as we forgive those who trespass against us.
And lead us not into temptation,
but deliver us from evil.
For Thine is the Kingdom, the Power and the Glory.
For ever and ever.
Amen.

The Great Invocation
Brought forth by Djwhal Khul in the Alice Bailey books
From the point of Light within the mind of God
Let Light stream forth into the minds of men.
Let Light descend on Earth.
From the point of love within the heart of God
Let Love stream forth into the hearts of men.
May Christ return to Earth.
From the centre where the Will of God is known
Let purpose guide the little wills of men –
The purpose which the Masters know and serve.
From the centre which we call the race of men
Let the plan of Light and Love work out
And may it seal the door where evil dwells.
Let Light and Love and Power restore the Plan on Earth.

Your Birth Prayer

How would you like to take your own unique mantras that have come from you inner journeying in the quantum inner fields and make them into divine prayer for your birth?

For Example:

I give all to the light
For the highest good of all beings
to know my baby births in beautiful divine flow,
Guided by light and love,
By the mother of love.
I just that she will hold me as I birth in the dance of light with my baby,
Happily, easily, comfortably.
We flow in the power of love
And my baby is born well,
Rejoicing in beauty and light.
Amen.

Feel the words on the inner, take them to the inner, and notice any blocks and if they are there revisit the inner to shift the blocks with Light until you absolutely align with your birth movie. Feelings, smelling, tasting the beautiful birth and if you wish you can set your prayer to music and as you listen to that music each say you feel the prayer manifesting in the Light.

Divine Mother, Birthing Goddess

The Goddess has 10,000 names, and throughout time and world traditions she has always existed in the form of Her many aspects. Cosmic Mother, Virgin Mary, Madonna, Mother Mary, Isis, Lady of Light, Blessed Virgin, Divine Mother, Queen of Angelic realms and Ascended Master, Goddess, Guide, Guru and Protector for birth and children. Mary is but one aspect of the Divine Goddess and you may choose to worship the Goddess in so many, many other forms.

Mer means beloved and derives fro the name for water and light. The Amun wives of Egypt were all Mers, or Marys. It is the sacred name for the Priestesses of the Goddess in Her many forms. Some say in Her original and first incarnated form manifest on Earth, She was Ma-Ra incarnated in Lemuria. Ma-Ra meaning "the Goddess who is the mother of the Sun". She is simply Divine Love. Ma Ra, the Divine Mother, is currently working with Lightworkers to re-empower women and bring back the Divine Feminine wisdom to earth.

It is essential that women re-find their power and enable men also to be free. The patriarchal attack on women has also disempowered all men. As mothers of sons and daughters, we teach our children how to become fully empowered men and women in the New Age. It is up to women to change the world. It is said that when all women return their menstrual blood to the earth (living and birthing in harmony with the earth and with Her flow) then the men will put down their weapons and come home.

Isis and Mary are names of different aspects of the Goddess. Ma Ra manifested as Isis during the reign of the mystery schools of Egypt. This soul is the feminine deity of the entire human race, the great Mother Deity of all Mankind is known as many names but belongs to no religious order. Her different names represent the different parts of her: the Divine Mother Goddess Ma Ra encompasses all of the following female beings of Light, but you can invoke different names to bring down the different elements that you require of the Goddess. For example, invoked as Isis, she brings you female power.

The Goddess power in Lemuria was known as "Ila". In Atlantis this power became "Ushas" and "Isis". After division set in and Atlantis was destroyed, the power of nurturing, the power of Divine Love, as a balance, was removed from civilisation. Now it is returning.

For humanity to heal itself and to thrive in the new dawn of Aquarius, we need to connect to the Divine Love again and bring in the female energy to balance this with the male - yin yang, sun moon, ida pingala, within each of us.

I highly recommend that men work with the Divine Mother as well as women, and likewise that women work with male deities too, in order to harmonise, access and align both parts of ourselves with each other. Through healing ourselves and birthing from a space connected to our inner God and Goddess aligned as one, we heal our planet and our future generations.

There is a meditation and more information on this in the section "Clear Connection" under finding your male / female balance, since to heal our female selves is also to heal our inner male.

What does the Divine Mother mean to you and how can you embody this principle for yourself as a Divine woman and as an empowered woman?

I invite you, if you are not doing so already, to really immerse into the many aspects of the Goddess. Look to her role, her worship, her ceremonies, her myths and traditions and get to develop a deep inner connection with Her. Perhaps you might buy a Goddess Tarot pack or go on a Goddess workshop. If you already have a very deep connection with Her, now is the time to go much deeper, whilst you are pregnant you are wide open and ready to receive her initiations. They will come to you in meditation, not through texts to read. Go sit with her and get to know her intimately for yourself and let her guide you. She is the one who will hold you when you birth, and the deeper you connect with her in your pregnancy, the more you will feel her in your birth.

For example, you may like to imagine her beautiful blue draping over and holding your baby, body, birth, pregnancy and children. You may call her Mother Mary (she has a special connection with children). You could make an offering to her by using special crystal such as aquamarine and watermelon tourmaline on a blue cloth. (Use the colours of fabrics and any other names of the Divine Mother Goddess that resonate for you). In your mind's eye see her blue silk enveloping you and say *"Mother Mary, I invoke you to hold and guide my pregnancy and birth, let it be filled and watched over by your guiding light, may you bless me and enable me to contact my inner divine goddess at the hour of my birth, may our birth be blessed by your light"*

Meditation on the Divine Mother

Find an image of the Divine Goddess or Mother that you love, and that embodies all the energies and colours of divine birth for you.

Place it in front of you with a candle set forward between the image and you. Dim or switch off all other lights. Go into meditation with your eyes closed and take many deep breaths in and out. Tune into the breath.

When you are ready, open your eyes and look at the image of the Divine Motherthat you have chosen. Feel the qualities of the image. As you tune into the vibration of the picture see the Mother guiding and protecting you now whilst pregnant, during your birth, and after the birth guiding you as a mother and your children.

Now see yourself as Divine Mother too. Embrace these qualities for yourself. Be a Divine Mother, and feel yourself as a Divine other within.

Keep breathing.

Please actually do this! Do this for 30 minutes or more.

You can bring this energy to you anytime simply by looking at this image and taking a few deep breaths. The Divine Mother is always there waiting for you.

Beings of Light for Help with Pregnancy and Childbirth

Many people believe that Beings of Light, especially Angels, are one with God and as such are neither male or female, like our own souls. Here they are listed as one or the other to represent the part of them to which we can tune in to and connect to. There are many Masters and Goddesses to help us and below are just a few for a suggestion for you to reflect upon and see which ones leap out for you. Chant these names to access immense power towards and within your birth and birthing manifestations. Find their images and place them in your birth room.

Masters and Beings of Light

Examples of Goddesses and masters that aid with pregnancy and children. These are just a few, the list is endless, she is after all the Goddess of 10,000 names.

Mary Magdalene - Female power. Mary Magdalene was as powerful as Jesus Christ and they worked together as Husband and Wife, King and Queen each as powerful as one another. Yin and yang, sun and moon. Like Jesus, she is a master.
Archangel Metratron - Crystal children.
Artemis - Protector, female power. Said to help with adoption and conception.
Aphrodite - Associated with feeling like a beautiful birthing woman.
Brigit - Female power and protection

Dana - Conception, parenting issues and twins.

Hathor - Conception, parenting issues and harmonious pregnancy.

Ishtar - Conception and parenting. Feminine power. Focus and clarity.

Isis - Female power

Diana - Pain free birth, protector.

Princess Diana - guides children in need.

Kwan Yin - Eastern form of Mother Mary, carrying the same energy as a protector of children

Lady Nada - Twin flame of Jesus, ascended master version of Mary Magdalene

Vista - Protector of children

Also - Venus, Tara, Giri Bala, Therese, Theresa of Avila, Guinevere, Sri Anandamayi Ma, Sri Saradamani Devi, Lady Portia, Goddess of Liberty, Lady Charity, Pallas Athena, Elizabeth, mother of John the Baptist, St Clare, Abundantia, St Catherine of Sienna (Helena Blavatsky and Joan of Arc in a previous incarnation), Sedan, Sulis. Mother Amma is alive today and travels the world to bring blessing and Light to all. You can meet her at one of her visits to your country for a blessing.

Goddesses from the Rose include Mother Mary, Isis, Artemis, Aphrodite, Qual Yin, White Buffalo Calf Woman, the Saint AnandaMayaMa, Venus, Black Madonna and Saint Sarah (both aspects of MM), Ameratsu, Kali Ma, Cailleach, Ixchel, Istar Star of Sirius & Inanna, Bridget, Rhiannon, Triple Goddess (maid, mother, crone), Mahaji (wife of Babaji), Sophia, Epona, Selena, Ceridwen, Coventina, Hekate, Devi, Aine, the Oracle at Delphi, the witch, ancient priestesses, your inner enchantress.

Her message and energy is also brought forward by Divine Masculine ascended masters, sages & prophets such as Jeshua Christ, Yogananda, Babaji, Lord Krishna, Lord Buddha, Lord Shiva, Ganesha, Saturn, Osirus, Horus, Archangel Micheal, Sanat Kumara, the Oak and the Holly Kings, Lugh, St Frances, Pan.

You may also like to work with the moon, the stars and galactics of Sirius, Pleiades, Venus and Andromeda and many more, including of course working primarily with Gaia. You can work with all the 5 elements, and especially the waters of the Mother and also with the different roses, your birthing shaman, your ancient midwife, your inner wild woman, other flowers and trees, Angels and elementals such as Fairies, animal guides, the great cosmic kundalini snake, the possibilities are endless and she comes in all these for and many, many more.....

The following list of Ascended Masters from the Great White Brotherhood has been selected from Joshua David Stone - "Master Kuthumi, Krishna, Rama, Adonis, Shakti, Lord Ganesha, Hanuman, El Morya, Djwal Khul, Saint Germain, Melchizedik (protection and crystal children), Metratron, Horis (mother son relationship), Yogananda, Babaji, Lahiri Mahasaya, Serapis Bey, Hilarion, Lord Maitreya, Paul the Venetian, Sanat Kumara, Vywamus, Buddha, Sai Baba, Baba Muktananda, Guru Nanak, Ramakhrishna, Ramana Marharshi , Maharaji, Ram Dass, Sri Aurobindo, Swami Vivekananda, Avalokitesvara, Patanjali, Osiris, Sandalphon, Enoch, Thoth, Appolonius of Tyanna, Shirdi SaiBaba, Sri Sankara, Swami Nityananda, Kabir, Confucius, Lao Tse, Mohammed, Mahavira, Meishu-Sama, Mahatma Ghandi, Sri Yukteswar, Helios, Zoraster, Pallas Athena, the Seven Mighty Elohim (Hercules, Apollo, Heros, Purity, Cyclopia, Peace, Arcturus), Archangels (as above), Mahatma, Avatar of Synthesisi, Allah Gobi, the Great Divine Protector, Melchior ... to name but a few!"

In the Golden Age all human beings are great masters like these - this is what it means to be a human-being - but we are currently diverted!

It is up to women to anchor the Divine Female essence and start to return us back to our true path. Pregnant women have huge power in their meditations to seed this Light upon Earth!

Jeshua the Christ and Mary Magdalene

Religious understandings of Mary seem are out of touch with cosmic truth, and used as a political tool to control and enslave people, or even worse, to murder and end any female Goddess practises - as seen in the mass murder of women in the witch hunts, attacks upon indigenous tribes and orders such as the mass murder of the cathar (the pure ones who followed Her ways). Many religions, which have their roots in sacred texts of truth, have been distorted for reasons of power, and disempowered women (and men) for centuries and this drove the Goddess worshippers into secrecy. I highly recommend the book 'Women with the Alabaster Jar' by Margaret Starbird for a fascinating understanding of how the Mer Goddess Light was secretly encoded into renaissance art.

Since the discovery of certain scrolls and the writing of certain key books by those with masonic knowledge (ie The Holy Blood and The Holy Grail by Michael Baigent, Richard Leigh and Henry Lincoln), Mary Magdalene is now finally being restored and understood to historically have been the equal to the guru Yeshua (Jesus) and to have worked together. When she was turned into a "whore", it was a great blasphemy, and we lost the Goddess energy on Earth. Male and female must be rebalanced now at this time. Like Yeshua, Mary was a prophet, healer and master and (so some authors such as Ralph Ellis have written and have attempted to prove) the true and rightful Queen of a great and powerful royal lineage from Rome, Mesopotamia and Egypt.

Jesus the Christ (Yeshua) was a master known as Jeshua Ben Joseph who became a channel for the Christ when he ascended. His spiritual partner and sister - wife was Mary Magdalene and together they anchored Divine Male and Female Light on Earth - Christ energy. When the Christian religion adopted him, for many reason the equal power and partner of the Magdalene energy was relinquished, which disempowered the true light of their message. Instead of focusing on the Light of the Christ, the proceeding religions chose instead to focus on the crucifixion, fears and sins of mankind. This brought the fear of God onto people, who needed the church to guide them. Women who practised herbal medicine and meditation were called witches and burnt alive (the word 'witch' comes from the words 'wicca' and 'wicked', which actually mean 'wise'). People could not own their power and worship God at home or in nature but instead had to go to church. There are still resonances from these beliefs around today in people's approaches to living, opinions, language and especially in people's beliefs about birth. Yet many people who carry this are not even conscious of it. People seem to be afraid of the wise women (witches) but not the ones who murdered her.

It was together with Mary that the master Jeshua Ben Joseph became a channel for the Christ Light, bringing it down to Earth. The return of Christ does not mean the return of this master, but a return of the Christ Light Consciousness that Jeshua and Mer channelled through together, it also signifies the Return of the Divine Feminine, so she may rise again and Her ancient and beautiful harmonious ways of the rose may once again be restored to grace.

Visualisation to Connect with your Spirit Guides and Goddesses

Close your eyes, relax. Take some deep breaths and keep on breathing deeply and slowly. Now return to your garden, your safe space. Down the stairs and through the door. Feel what it is like to be there.

Once you feel ready and have explored and dwelt there a while, go to your chair and rest.

Now it is time to ask your spirit guides and God's helpers to come and be present. You have already connected to your birthing guides in the previous visualisations, but now you are asking to connect to any other guides and Goddesses. There may also be more birthing beings from angelic and spirit world who want to come forward and connect to you, or it may be the same one(s).

Be still and see who comes.

You may imagine or get a sense of the names and people or beings, what they look like or how they dress, or this may not be important. You may just feel a sense of presence beside you. They may be male or female or completely androgynous. They may be orbs or grids, or trees. You can also ask specific beings, who you feel drawn to, if they will come to you now. Communicate with them. Ask for signs and calling cards.

Those who come to you will always be Beings of light since you have asked for light and you are in your sacred garden. Keep connecting. A Being of light is just that - a being full of Light and Love… they talk only from a place of unconditional love and they never judge nor compare.

Spend time just being with any who come to you. Don't try too hard to talk or get messages, just be there with them, just connecting, just being.

You may like to ask for blessing and healing, as well as seals of completion, before giving thanks and coming back. They may give you a special gift that means something to you.

Finally imagine and focus on the Divine Mother energy again: imagine the goddess as you see her, in front of you and become her. Really take on Her energy and become the Goddess in the form that she comes, if it feels right to do so. This is called blending, to let Her overLight you, and something that you may like to do in birth. She is here to help and guide you through the heart, and is happy for you to take on her energy in your heart for your deepest happiness as you are a child of Goddess.

When you feel filled with the Goddess in your heart and connected to your beautiful birthing spirits, it is time to come back.

Come back to the room through the door and up the stairs. Give thanks and feel that you are now guided for the highest good of all concerned! So be it and so it is!

Using Colour

Use colour to cleanse, protect and relax in pregnancy and birth by imagining it surrounding you and breathing it in and out to the place where you need it most. You can use your intuition to *find your own colours* for use in meditation, refer to the list below, or look into chakras. You can find out more elsewhere about chakras, but the simple list here is for quick reference in relation to pregnancy and birth. In the actual birth you may be surprised by which colours come. Be open.

Strength and Holding - Gold
Cleansing - White
Safety of Archangel Micheal - Deep blue cloak
Grounding (base) - Red roots from feet deep into earth's centre
Lower abdomen comfort - Orange (a good colour to birth from if you experience pain in the abdomen)
Power and empowerment (solar plexus) - Yellow
Compassion (heart) - Emerald green
Baby love and protection (centre chest) - Pink
Creative communication, connection (throat) - Turquoise blue
Psychic insight (third eye) – Indigo - sit inside a sparkling indigo temple
God and spirit connection (crown) - Violet and gold

Two Colour Visualisations

Pink and Blue Mother Mary Visualisation for Baby Holding and Connection

Close your eyes and imagine a figure of 8 around you and your baby and/or child. The part of the eight that encircles you is blue and the part around your baby is pink. This will keep you held by the Goddess Mary energy, safe, in love and connected. It will also keep your baby and you clear in your own spheres. You can also put the figure of 8 around you and your baby in a golden sphere of light for further holding and alignment.

For more than one child, do it more than one time, rather than putting them all in one circle of the 8, or else imagine a spiral like an eight around all of you, so that each one of you is in a circle on your own yet connected. Imagine the flow around all of you, connecting and swirling around you all as one infinite line; blue around the parents and pink around the children.

You can draw this out on paper as well.

Colour Visualisation for Birthing Comfort

You may like to ask for a colour to come in to the birth space as you birth and then breathe it in and out to your belly to help you birth and ease any sensation that needs it. The colour that comes may surprise you.

Or imagine a beautiful rainbow flowing all around you and breathe in each of the beautiful colours. Do this regularly throughout pregnancy to prepare you for the birth. You can do this every morning as part of your daily pregnancy morning ritual. Try it now.

Rays

Like the chakra colours, there are many different and new Light rays that are currently entering our planet to help us at this time of change. They are all aspects of God's personality, and are like working with the different colours of a rainbow or the different aspects and forms of the Goddess. They are emanations from Light Source.

Reiki is a type of healing Light ray. Today there are many different strands of Reiki:. The more traditional ones are Angelic, Karuna, Seichem and Usui, and now there are many more including my own channelled Rose Reiki, Dolphin Reiki, Aphrodite Reiki and so forth. There are different ways of teaching and differing types of initiations. Originally Dr. Usui the founding master taught with just three initiations.

Another form of rays are the seven major rays of 'God Virtue'. These are akin to the 7 chakras and 7 gates. They all need each other, too much of one leads to imbalance. They are equally balanced to be male and female. To embrace and invite and work with all seven of them is to become in full power with the seven aspects of God.

Other types of rays include the twelve Ascended Master rays, the 7 Gem Rays (silver, gold, platinum, ruby, emerald, sapphire, and diamond), the Violet flame, the Mahatma energy, Angelic and Crystal rays, Celestial Rays. Vortex healing rays… to name but a few.

Many masters have their own rays and colours. For example, Mary Magalene can come both as a spirit guide as well as as a consciousness. She often brings the magenta ray as well as the lavender violet.

When you are pregnant you are very open, so ask for spirit guidance before going to see someone. I wanted to attend an Angelic Ray initiation when I was pregnant, but for some reason I had some hesitation about it. I felt like I was forcing it. I put out a prayer for guidance to the universe. Two days before it was due to start, the lady rang to tell me it was cancelled.

Example Exercise to Invoke Light Rays

Close your eyes and take breaths.
Ground with red roots and ask for holding.
Now ask the ray that you intend to work with to come forwards. One may surprise you or you may have one in mind already. Get a sense of it. Breathe it in. Swirl it around you. Send it to your birth and to your baby.

Some rays need to be transmitted by a teacher and lineage and you need to go and seek your teacher out to connect into the lineage in person, for example in some types of yoga and Reiki the ray radiates from the guru connection, from teacher to teacher. Other times you can connect directly yourself and do not need to go to a teacher or guide unless you want to.

The Venus Ray

The power of this ray is unconditional love, to open your heart to the light. You can be initiated into this ray in your crown, heart and feet chakras and then use it for healing, or simply ask before going to sleep or in meditation for initiation on a soul level.

The Violet Flame Of Transmutation

Whilst you can use the colours blue, white and gold for protection, the colour violet can be used for purifying and healing/changing. You can invoke the violet ray by saying
"I am a master. Through divine Light and Grace I now invoke the Violet flame to transmute the energies in and around [me/the planet/the birth/the baby/the sensation etc] and to transform them into light. Let it be so. So it is".

Imagine it swirling around you as you already have done with the White Christ Light.

The Silver Violet Flame

This ray will transform negative energy into something more beautiful. You can call upon St Germain or Archangel Zadkiel to surround any thought or situation that needs transforming in order for your healthy dream birth to occur, for the highest will and good of all concerned.

Think about it, visualise it, imagine it, sense it or invoke it mentally by saying "*I invoke the silver violet ray to heal anything that stands in the way of my perfect birth, to heal any situation that may block our perfect birth, to purify my body ready for birth, to go to the right places in my body and heal anything that may need healing in order to birth easily and smoothly and well, to heal any discomfort in the birth place now, to blaze a trail in front of me to purify my imminent birth…*"

The flame includes the colours from lavender, through lilac to deepest violet.

Angel Healing

Angels work through the heart so you must open your heart to heal. Angels are God's helpers, and exist in every religion and spiritual practise under differing names. Some people see them as men and women with wings, others as grids or orbs or colours. They will help with anything if you ask them to. **But you must ask**. (Remember when you pray you do so without affirming lack and need but by affirming abundance in the positive and but affirming it is so). Simply say "*Angels, please help with my birth to be flowing with ease and comfort…I invoke the qualities of …..*" then let go and know that it is being taken care of.

Visualisation for Angelic Healing

Focus on the part of you that needs the healing, or on the birth that you want. Then breathe deeply and breathe in angelic healing light. This is golden.
Ground yourself (and the person you are healing if you are healing another)
To ground: Imagine roots from your feet going into the centre of the earth to ground you. Feel the Earth's energy coming back to you.
Ask for holding and imagine white light surrounding you.
Invoke the angels. Imagine a column of golden angelic light coming from the universe and entering your crown chakra, attuning you to the higher energies. Hold your hands up and ask three times that the angels allow you to be a pure channel for healing. Feel their loving presence around you. Ask them to fill your hands with gold. You now have golden healing hands.

Place your hands where you feel you need it after a body scan. Connect with your feet last. Alternatively, send the energy to your birth and to your baby. This is a very powerful healing.

Smooth the aura three times at the end, thank the angels for their help and drink water.

Be aware that children and animals need less time, and watch out for any healing crisis where symptoms feel worse as they leave the body.

Clear Channel of Light Meditation

Close your eyes and relax.
Notice but don't change your breathing.
Ask for grounding.
Keep breathing.
Imagine red roots from your feet going deep into the centre mother earth.
Breathe the light from the earth up into your feet and up through your legs into your tummy.
Fill your tummy up with the Earth's light.
When you feel grounded, imagine a light from a glowing divine star pouring down from the sky into your head and into your heart.
When you feel this clearly, bring the Earth energy up to your heart and let it mingle there.
Now bring the Earth energy up higher to your head and out whilst bringing the starlight down to the ground and into the Earth from your feet.

You are now a clear channel for the world. Shine and radiate the love from your heart to the world and to your baby.
I am clear, I am light, I am love, I am a clear channel of light, for the highest good of all concerned, so be it and so it is! Amen.

Start using this daily in your pregnancy and use it in your birth if you like: what a wonderful, clear place to birth from!

Visualisation to connect with your baby's soul:

(You can connect with your baby using the Temple of Power Visualisation, as well as the one here. Use it whenever you want to communicate or find your baby's soul, even after the birth for Intuitive Connected Parenting.)

First rub your belly and talk to your baby.
Imagine your baby is happy and radiant.
Listen to any message that your baby might want to give you or any voices you might feel.
Ask for protection for the two of you.
Now imagine that there is a flight of beautiful stairs spread before you. These are the stairs that lead to the spirit land of your baby's soul.
Walk down them and find yourself in the most beautiful green field full of wild flowers. There are rich green trees around, the sun is hot but there is a warm breeze and it is dappled by the leaves in the lovely trees. There are mountains in the distance. This is a protected safe spot which means that there is nothing here that can harm you. This is a place of purity and love. It is protected by white light.

Make your intention clear: you would like to connect to your baby's soul.

As you walk, you will come across a river. This river leads to the land of unborn souls. See a boat and a guide. Enter the boat and sit with your guide as you cross the river. Who is your guide? Is it dark or light, silent, still? Is there a waterfall? Do you pass it?

When you arrive at the shore and leave the boat, you see that in front of you is a beautiful mountain. You climb the mountain and at the top, near the clouds, you find spirit.

Here float high resonating angelic Beings of Light. Fill up with their light and ask your baby's spirit to come forth if he or she has not already done so.

She or he may come down from a rainbow of light, a star, or be waiting silently for you on the mountain top. See this Being and ask for his or her name if you want. Ask for messages from your baby, or just be with them. They may communicate with you or they may not. This could be a moment to also get some information for the birth, but mainly it is about simply just being and enjoying connection.

Get a sense of their guides, these are guides that can help you in the birth space too and help you with protection as your child grows. You have probably already met them in previous visualisations in this book.

When it is time, leave your beautiful child on this island of love and light and return across the river on the boat where your guide awaits you.

Thank your child and see them protected. Hug them. Let them know that they are deeply loved by you and that you are looking forward to meeting them and receiving them when it is their time to cross the river into your arms and the world of form. Your child may wave to you.

On the day of birth they will be crossing this river to come to you in the dreamland of form. You could imagine this as you birth.

You only need to do this meditation once, it is very powerful, but it may stay with you and you may keep returning to it if it feels right to do so. For example, even after the birth, you can close your eyes and imagine your child's spirit on this island, letting you hear them clearly: "No! Broccoli is not right for me!" " You can also use the method below to communicate with your baby, or find your own way of connecting with their Higher Self.

Return through the garden and give thanks.
Ground and protect.
You have now met the soul of your child for the highest good of all concerned.

My baby grows in light. My womb is full of light and I am a womb-an of light!

So be it and so it is for the highest good of all! Amen!

Ceremony

Ceremony plays an important part in clearing the spirit in preparation for birth and in welcoming your baby. Ritual and ceremony use the same six principles as prayer. This ceremony is the culmination and final prayer in your daily pregnancy ritual. When you turn all your mantras, inner healing and journal exercises into prayer and then take that prayer to ceremony, it becomes even more powerful. Ensure your intention, thoughts, dedications and so on are pure and clear. Use the following as a guide.

The Birth Manifestation Ceremony
Taking your prayer to ceremony

Go to a special place of power at an appropriate time, alone or with your birthing partner(s)/children. You may return to this place to bury your placenta. Have your prayer to hand. Take candles, wear special clothing, bring images and flowers and so forth. Make this very special. make it a beautiful ritual. Choose a special day. You might like to honour the 4 elements of fire, earth, air, water, and the 4 directions before you commence.

Then see yourself in a sphere of golden light. Ground yourself with red roots, growing deep into the Earth.

Start clearly by invoking the presence of the spiritual beings to whom you are most drawn, asking them to be present with you. You can also invoke rays or energies that you wish to be present with you in your birth. See the colours and Beings come down and swirl around you.

Read out your prayer, your birthing manifestation sheet and birth rehearsal.

Ask these beings to make this happen in whatever ways they can/however they can, for the highest good of all concerned.

Ask them to guide and watch you from now onwards so that everything that happens helps to create this positive birth.

Ask them to help you to hear them in times of confusion and fear, so that you may follow their guidance clearly.

Ask them to send messages to you that you can hear and follow.

Ask them to watch over and to protect your birth and your birthing family and baby.

Give thanks. For the highest good of all concerned, know that your birth is in the process of manifestation.
So be it and so it is!

Be clear when you have finished your ceremony. Pay attention to and follow any intuitive feelings that may follow your ceremony, like going over to the nearby stream and washing your face. Ground yourself when it is finished and close the space. After you have done this ritual you now know that it is so. Your prayer has been taken by Goddess in the ceremony and from now onwards every single thing that happens, no matter whether it appears to be good luck or bad luck, is a part of a series of events in holding you and this prayer. You might like to also affirm "this or something better". Because at the end of the day, always remember the universe may have an even higher plan. So don't force…. allow….

About This Ceremony

As I have mentioned, you can wear special clothing, colours and crystals, and play special music and chants. If you want to, you can use the five elements (water earth, fire, air, ether). You can do this on a special day or holy day/number or moon phase, which can make it infinitely more powerful. Use water, flowers as offerings, feathers, ring bells singing bowls and read words of wisdom, if you feel like it.

It is your ritual.

From now onwards you can be assured that your birth will be divine in whatever shape or form it takes for the highest good of all concerned. So be it and so it is!

From now onwards, let go but keep on following the energy – only see people and go to places that "hum"/resonate for you.

Be discreet about this ceremony. Keep your ritual place quiet, it is between you and those who are there. Ensure that anyone who is with you for the ritual is there to support you and believes in what you are doing, and that you have discussed it beforehand, so that it is your ceremony together. This is a private, sacred ceremony, and it is most powerful when it is kept as a quiet and sacred truth so I highly recommend just doing it alone or with your beloved or both.

It is particularly important not to share your personal rituals with people who do not believe in the power of them. The spiritual Beings can never be diminished but your ability to hear and believe in them could be damaged if you have your beliefs questioned by those who don't understand them. If you want to, you can keep on connecting to these beings regularly in your own home by just closing your eyes, connecting, talking and giving thanks.

When you are in the birthing space you may forget to tune into these beings and that is fine because you have now already invoked them in preparation. However, you may wish to create a reminder for yourself or ask your birthing partner to remind you to do so. You could ask as your birth begins for them to be present and to guide you and protect you and give you clear messages throughout the birth. Your birth partner could have a signal or touch that you associate with your angels and that can reconnect you in the birth. Think of one right now!

If you feel intimidated by medical advisors or confused in drama type situations, you can ask your spiritual guides to take over. Medical staff usually do not treat birth as a sacred. You could ask your birthing spiritual Beings to come to you to give clear guidance, then tell your medical health advisor that you need ten minutes to be alone (or just go to the toilet). This gives you time alone just to tune in. Ask for a sign. They know what is for the best and will make it happen. After all, it might be that it is right for you to be induced. You just follow the energy.

There is another ritual designed for welcoming your baby and burying the placenta in the birth chapter.

Creating Sacred Space for Pregnancy and Birth

Your birth environment is one of the key aspects to attaining the birth you want. Use the protection visualisation and the one below to clear it so that only supportive things, events, and people are present.

Also do what you can physically to make it beautiful. Whether you decide to birth at home or not, you are spending your pregnancy at home so create a beautiful energised space in which to grow your baby and replenish your soon-to-be birthing body. Your home is your sanctuary. If you do not have your own home or you share it with others, then do what you can to make your own space clear within it.

Make use of the nesting instinct to **calmly** clear out your house – everything that has a negative vibration must go. Keep going through book cases and cupboards and cleanse or get rid of anything that feels like it has a stagnant vibe, passing as much as possible on to a charity or recycling centre.

If you want, use this time to buy or create beautiful new things that make you feel abundant. You are a child of God, therefore you deserve abundance. Make your home a temple. Use Feng Shui or simply your own instincts.

You do not need to acquire anything else if you do not want to, but simply fill your home with light. Instead of bringing home all the baby-clutter that many magazines will suggest you need, create a clear and positive, harmonious, vibrating home. This is the most important thing your baby needs.

Music is really important. Play and listen to uplifting spiritual music and chanting to clear your house. Use crystals and plants and the power of your mind – imagine your home vibrating in a clear and positive protective light bubble.

Think about which objects will enable you to be in a sacred space during the birth?

Candles; water; chanting music; incense; oil burners; smudging; a beautiful birth ball; crystals to hold and place around the room (especially rose quartz); oils for you and your baby; potions; herbs and homeopathic kits to hand for the birth; beautiful clothing, dressing gown or loose shirt; comfortable furnishings and blankets for afterwards or a sacred cloth to drape over your baby. Will you birth in front of your altar and all the images and sacred objects that you have placed there? Will you place a postcard or image that inspires you in other rooms in case you end up in there? What will you pack to take with you in case you go anywhere else? Do note that if you end up going to hospital and cannot take anything with you… they are only props and the truth is in your heart. You really need nothing but God.

Visualisation for Sacred Space

Close your eyes and go down into a relaxed space taking deep and relaxed breaths. Letting go. Relaxing.

When you have reached it, imagine the place where you are currently living in front of you. This is where you are growing your baby.

See the door in front of you and get a sense of the door handle being a hand that you are going to reach out and touch. As you do so, what do you feel? Give your home light and healing. Open the door and note the first sensations you pick up on. Give light to the room into which you walk and look round it, placing light wherever it needs it. Now into the next room and the next… go all around your house, take time to go around every room and cupboard, noting and placing light where it is needed.

Thank and bless your house for holding and protecting you.

Coat it in a protective shield of light and colour. See the colours of love. Ask a guardian angel to spread her/his wings around the house and keep it safe.

Whoever enters your house from now on will be enveloped in this light and people who are not wanted will no longer come near.

Now go into your birth space: either revisit it again in this house or go elsewhere. Sit and be in that space and get a sense of it and feel if it needs anything. Give the space healing and light where it needs it. Now ask your birth angels to heal this space and fill it with light so that it may support you in your birth. Let the space fill with deep Christ-light and colours of warmth and protection. Ask if you need to place any crystals anywhere. Whenever you are in this space now, you will feel the light, protection and radiance that emanates from it. Ask a guardian angel to spread his/her wings around the birth space.
Now see a protective shield of light and colour surrounding the space. Whoever enters your birthing space from now on will be enveloped in this light and people who are not wanted will no longer come near.

Bless and thank both spaces and know now that for the highest good of all concerned, your home and birth space are blessed!

So be it and so it is!

5 - Clear Connection

Connect only with people who believe that you can do it.

"The energy and consciousness that is in the birthing room very much influences how the birth will proceed."
Valerie J Taylor, midwife.

Connecting with Yourself

Use the visualisation below to connect with your own power and yourself at any time before or during the birth process. You can use this to connect with your baby too. The need for self-nourishment and self-love cannot be emphasised strongly enough. Keep on practising this Higher Self connection to support and carry you beyond the birth and through the parenting years.

Temple of Power Visualisation

Everyone has a throne of power in the higher realms where they sit to connect with their Higher Self and inner power. Find yours and you can sit there whenever you need to fill yourself with strength and inner power. You can also go and sit there to communicate with Higher Beings, your children's souls, or to get information whenever you need it.

Close your eyes and take deep breaths. Relax fully. Really take the time to do so and when you feel totally relaxed, go to your beautiful safe place. Now ask for a tunnel to appear that will take you to your Temple of Power. Walk along it and find a door to your Temple of Power. As you enter the door, notice what it looks like and what the temple is like. Enter the temple and see a throne in front of you. This is your throne and your seat of power. What does it look like? Is it inside or outside? Take some time to let the image come to you and really get a sense of where it is and what it looks like.

Now go over to your throne and be seated. What does it feel like to sit in your power? Take time to sit there and enjoy the feeling. Fill with Light and fill with power. Whenever you feel needy, come here to fill up with Light and strength. Take at least 5 minutes now in silence to dwell in your seat of power…This is the main part of this meditation so really feel this space and this temple.

Now when you are ready, you can ask some guides of Light to come to talk with you. Invite them to you and see what messages they have for you.

If you want to continue to do so, you can use this space to talk with your child's Higher Soul. Invite the soul to come and state your intention, asking for the highest good of all and with the highest respect. See what comes. The gender may be clear, or not (try not to fixate on this but instead see a be-ing), perhaps you may see how the soul is dressed, hear what they say, or just get a vague sense of who they are. Does he or she have any messages for your parenting skills or any birthing requests? Why have they chosen you as their parent? Why are they coming?

When you are ready, you can go on to connect with other future children or with the souls of previous ones who never were born. You can also connect with the spirits of children who are already in form to check in and see if they have any parenting requests or needs.

When it is right to do so, thank them and return to yourself.

Keep filling with Light in your throne.

When you are completely full you may return through the door, closing it behind you, go up the tunnel, to your safe place and back to your body wherever you may be.

Relax and trust in any messages that have come to you.

I am in my fullness of power for the highest good of all.
So be it and so it is!
Amen!

Connecting with your Baby

There are many visualisations in this book to help with connecting with your baby.

Make sure you make time every day to connect with your baby by rubbing oils into your belly and womb at the same time as talking to your baby and affirming positive mantras. Fill your baby and your body up with Light as you do this. You may want to roll your hips and move with the self massage saying things like "I turn birthing over to you, my beautiful baby and to you my beautiful body". Imagine your baby in pure Light, a picture of health and happiness. Get yourself into a space by listening and relaxing to music that makes you feel full of love and euphoric. Then send the love signals to your unborn baby, and keep on doing so throughout the days. Constantly tune into LOVE.

At times, you may want to reflect on how you feel about the conception of your baby and heal any issues that may lurk there. Take your time to really connect to your baby as a Being, not as a gender. Thinking about the gender of a baby can take up a tremendous amount of energy, and whilst it can be fun to think about it (and impossible not to, at times) take care to also ensure you tune into your baby as a Being. Likewise if you do know the gender of your baby, keep connected to the Being, not the gender.

You might like to take some time to imagine that you are your baby. What does it feel like? What do you need more of? This is something you can do after your baby is born, as they are growing up.

Use this as a time of practise for tuning in and giving over to your body. Practise resting in the silence between thoughts.

Connecting with your Birth Supporters

It is important to find the right support in order to create the relaxed vibe that you want and need in the birth space.

The importance of the role of your birthing partner(s) cannot be emphasised strongly enough. Birthing partners are the people who are there to support and **protect your space so that you can let go and relax in birth**.

If you want your partner present, now is the time to clear any relationship issues so that you can birth in clarity together. Your birthing partner has to be someone you can trust absolutely. Both you and your partner fulfil the role of both protector *and* birthing shaman since modern midwives are mostly unable to perform this role. You could look into finding other support such as an Independent Midwife, friend, doula or alternative practitioner, or you may feel connected enough to your Higher Self that you do not feel that you need external support. Perhaps you know someone who is not birth-aware but is sacred-aware, who might want to be present as a guide for a sacred birth.

Your birth supporters include your partner, midwives, doctors, babysitters, cleaners, food angels, family, friends; it includes *all* the people who are present around your time of birth to help to make it easier. Their role is to support **your** birthing wishes. They are there to help you to create what you want. Use the manifestation action plan to help find the right people to appear at the right time for you and your baby. Treat yourself to a cleaner and a food angel for a while. This is your female birthing right. In ancient cultures, mothers are massaged and looked after for forty days after giving birth.

Your birth supporter's key role, whoever they are, is to support you in your beliefs and desires, to be there and believe in you.

Remember that birthing itself is an intimate dance and anyone present is sharing in this intimacy. As already discussed, it is hard to have a sacred intimate birth with unfamiliar others present in the room as it can make you self conscious.

Very few midwives are able to support a sacred birth due to the health and safety standards they must legally follow, standards which often draw the birthing woman out of her trance state. The two often contradict. For example, in the U.K. observation during birth must legally take place. Being observed by someone may mean that you feel watched and invaded at some level. Can you imagine being observed whilst making love or emptying your bowels?

Think about your expectations concerning birth supporters.

Both you and your partner need to ask questions such as:

What are your expectations of your birth supporter's role in the birth space?
How could he/she be there for you, believing in you?
What qualities do you need in the birth from him/her?
What expectations does your Midwife have?
What do you expect of your Midwife?
What do you expect from yourself?
Can you let go and trust that the universe will manifest the right midwife for you at the right time, if you affirm this in your mantras?

"What each woman needs to do in labour reflects her individuality. "Natural Labour" means doing what comes naturally, for you…I feel the most important thing the birthing woman does is to listen to her own body and find out what her body is telling her she needs to do. And that neither the partner nor the midwife, nor the doula or whomever, should be giving orders, "now do that" because that interferes with what she is really trying to get from her body"

Marsden Wagener M.D.

The Birth Shaman is an ancient midwife who helps guide spirits to cross over the river from the otherworld.

Soul shamans exist in many ancient cultures, guiding people in the other direction – to die peacefully. Ram Dass talked about a concept call "dial – a – death", allowing those at the end of their lives to contact a person who understands their philosophy of life to help guide them to die consciously.

"You could die in a Christian metaphor, a Buddhist metaphor, a Muslim metaphor, whatever. There would be people from every tradition and we would do all we could to have every tradition represented: Wiccan, Zoroastrian, Rastafarian, you name it. That is, we would do our best to arrange whatever setting the die-er felt would maximise his or her chance of being turned inward towards God at the moment of death"
Paths to God, Living the Bhagavad Gita by Ram Dass

I dream of the same supportive and loving situation for birthing families, to help incarnating spirits arrive gently in a wonderful warm birth. Wouldn't it be wonderful if we were able to have Birthing Shamans to guide us into a trance state with mantra and herbs and incense, instead of midwives with paper work?

If it is not possible or desirable to have a Birth Shaman present in your birth, you can connect to and invoke one from the other worlds.

Invoking your Birth Shaman
What would your birthing shaman/ancient midwife do? How would she be?

Christa wrote in her birthing journal:

A wise, old woman who quietly leaves our family alone in our intimacy, enabling me to be alone to birth in my own power, simultaneously supporting us and me to do this, with her presence simply holding the space... either in the room or without, depending on her sensitive and intuitive responses to my vibes. At times she mops my face, strokes my hair, massages my shoulders whilst wafting incense around, guiding me to follow my instincts and be in my power to make it my birth by leading me into myself to follow my instincts at times when I may go into my head and leave my instincts behind. She responds to the vibes with whatever is needed at every moment, silent. Maybe she would not be in my room during the birth but sitting honourably in her own space elsewhere in the house. She is in a trance herself, guiding me (us) from the other side, in connection with all our family. When our baby is born, she is there supporting me to welcome and hold and feed our baby myself, and to cut my baby's cord if it feels right for me to cut it. She does this very sensitively, allowing time and space to flow in its own way. She does not take over and do it for me. She does not mop up the blood but lets me sit in it, absorbing it, grounded and earthed. She guides me in those precious, sacred first few weeks of becoming a mother, silently – from a distance – but is there for words of wisdom and head massages when I most need them. She would also be there for Paul and our relationship to help us both make the shift into becoming parents, and especially to help support him in the birth whilst he fulfils his role of protector and father.

Write out your vision of the perfect birthing shaman for you and invoke her/him to be present with you in the ether, someone whom you can imagine guiding you when you need the guidance.

The following invocation for an ancient midwife can be done in pregnancy as a birth preparation exercise, or in the birth space itself for guidance.

Invocation For Your Ancient Midwife

You have already communicated with some of your birthing spirits. In the Protection Exercise you invoked a birthing guide, and in the exercise for Connecting to Spiritual Beings, you communicated with your birthing angels. These birthing spirits are present with you now, and they are relevant here as you once again re-connect to invoke your Birth Shaman.

Close your eyes, relax and breathe.

Ground using the visualisation of roots from your feet and shine the white Light in and around you.

Enter your garden and go to your chair as before. This will be very familiar now.

Ask your birthing guide and angelic beings to come and be present again.
Thank them for being there and communicate with them if you wish or else just sit and be with them. Imagine any colours and get a sense of them.

Really enjoy the glorious feelings and sensations that you may get with them. Perhaps you tingle all over in their beauty.

Now ask for your Birth Shaman to come forward. This may be a birth guide or an angel or it may be someone completely new who works alongside them as a team.

Choose your midwife/shaman and get to know her (him/it). What does she look like? How does she sound? What does she have to say?

Connect and work with her, bring her wisdom to you to guide your birth and call to her in your birth space.

When you are ready and you have deeply connected with your spirit midwife, ask and invoke people who are present with you in your birth to be the right people for you at the right time.

Finally you can also focus on becoming Goddess energy and Divine Mother within, if you want to fill yourself up with the Goddess in your heart – imagine Her in front of you and fill yourself up with her Light, or imagine the image on the back of this book. Perhaps your birth shaman is the Divine Mother herself, or the Goddess within.

Give thanks and return through the door and up the stairs, keeping the Goddess in your heart and the connection with your birth shaman.

From now onwards if you want to, you can contact and work with this being, alongside other spiritual helpers and your own Higher Self, for any birth issues. Alternatively, it may be that connecting only once is necessary.

For the highest good of all concerned, my birthing shaman is now guiding my pregnancy and birth, so be it and so it is!

Connecting with your Birth Partner

(Note - I refer to your birth partner here as a "him", but the following is applicable to whoever your birth partner may be)

Do you want a birth partner? Are you sure you want it to be your partner (husband)?

You need to ask yourself this question, and not assume that your husband/partner should be there. Some men may be uncomfortable, which you will pick up on. If your man is uncomfortable, how does that make you feel? You need to heal any resentment. Your choices and decisions need to be based on positive feelings rather than negative situations. You may prefer a friend, doula or parent, or even to be unassisted with back up around if needed. Whilst making your choice about this, refer to the section later - What if your birth partner cannot support you?

If you decide you do not want any supporter there at all but want a totally unassisted childbirth, this should be a decision based on a happy and positive feeling with no resentment at all. The case for an unassisted childbirth is outlined in *Unassisted Childbirth* by Laura Kaplan Sanley. As discussed in this book, many people feel invaded during birth by having others present in the same space, and it can be hard to create a sacred birth with clinical strangers around you.

Isabel enjoyed an unassisted birth after consciously deciding to go for this during her third pregnancy. She had focused on following forgiveness exercises from previous births and, as she did so, she healed herself and realised she wanted to prepare herself for an unassisted home birth by the sea in her beach house. After researching and preparation, when she went into birth she was able to enjoy several days of going in and out of sensations with orgasm and gentle stimulation and self massage with olive oil. She felt fulfilled, happy and joyful, as she had come to realise during her pregnancy meditations that this was what she truly desired and felt right. It was an empowered decision from a positive place. Her partner and children were sometimes present in the house but left her to her own devices. They had signals set up should she require their presence. After two huge pulses and a membrane release in the bath she realised she was closer to birthing than she had thought and decided she wanted her children there. They woke up and came just in time as her baby slipped out easily onto the floor, her perineum completely intact.

If you do decide to do it alone, do your research and begin from an empowered, positive and prepared place like Isabel. Likewise, if you decide to have a birth partner, do the research and work together. What is the main role for your birth partner? Often your partner is there to protect your space so that you can relax and let go. You need absolute trust in him to be able do this.

Your partner's role is essential to your sacred birth. He is the yang sun energy and you are the yin moon energy and you birth together as sun and moon. Many men say they feel "helpless" in the birth space but your man can come into his power by sharing in the birth and birthing *with* you (even if this means from a different room) and protecting your trance space.

In the birth, your partner and anyone else present is there primarily to help keep you in your power, to stop you going into your head and keep you in your trance, in tune with your instincts. He can provide you with all your needs in the birthing space and, if you have rehearsed everything together previously, you can totally surrender and relax into the birth, knowing that he will sort anything out in the physical world. He is there to *protect* your space from unwelcome visitors and ensure that everything you need and want is provided for. He can also interpret changing situations according to previous preparations to improvise in the moment. He is there to support you to be in a safe and intimate meditative space. Trust is essential. Don't hand your power or blame over to him though, you are equally responsible and you both have to trust in God.

In the pregnancy, he can create and manifest the birth with you by doing his own manifestation work as well as sharing your own mantras with you. Whilst you do your practise alone with your baby on a daily basis, you also need to create time together to do birth rehearsals and meditations as outlined below.

Ways that your Birth Partner can Support you

1. by working together to fill the relationship with Light & Joy
2. by connecting with you as an empowered divine woman
3. by connecting with himself as an empowered divine man
4. by preparing the birth space with you and sharing the birth with you

"You deserve a lover who "seeks, cherishes, honours and delights in an empowered woman." The Love You Deserve, Scott and Shannon Peck

1. By Working Together to Fill the Relationship with Light & Joy

Relationships are fantastic karmic lessons in oneness!

It is essential that you feel totally at ease in your relationship with your birth partner/father of your child to birth well with them, **whether they are present in your life/the birth or not.** You want to create a relationship container that is held and glowing with Light with the father of your child, wheat you are with them still or not, as the birthing mother you need to feel good about it and them. If they are fully absent then you need to come to a place of peace and acceptance with this.

It is essential that your feelings are loving towards your children's father, not just for a tension-free birth, but since your relationship is the foundation for your baby and your future children. This is whether you are together or not, whether he is present or absent - the relationship means - how you feel about him within you, as the birthing mother. Your children will mirror all emotions that you and your partner have for each other and will draw upon this subconsciously as the basis for forming their developing personalities and characters. If you are no longer together, you need to heal your feelings about this with forgiveness and acceptance and release all resentments and hurts you may be carrying around so that you feel emotionally clear within yourself.

Use Part One to resolve anything that is bothering you and to find peace, acceptance and forgiveness with your partner/the father of your children.

By working on yourself and becoming full in your own power, and by giving to yourself what you most need and want in a partner, you will find your relationship starts to mirror your internal space.

Examples of Relationship Mantras

If problems are occurring in your relationship, for example bickering, or your partner does not treat you as you would like, or there is resentment about childcare, then you need to stop and ask yourself where the root of it lies. Ask questions such as "is our love a form of attachment?" "Do I have unrealistic expectations?" "What belief / emotion is the root cause of my resentment and what can I do about it?" You can go to Part One and tune into the inner subconscious belief pattens and traumas to connect, heal and then form a new vibration with a mantra that is aligned to the inner quantum healing work.

So the invite is to bring yourself to a place of full power with your source as yourself (or Goddess) using the meditations in this book. Then use mantra and apply the mantra to all persons.

So for example, if you feel unheard, begin by going within to connect to the inner trauma where you first ever felt unheard, when that was, what age you were, what that trauma looks like, what its true message is, and then bring the light into it to transform it into something else. That will lead to a new belief aligned to the new healing work that comes for within. As you start listening to yourself you may then affirm words form the new feelings that manifest, such as: "*I love and listen to myself, I am present with myself, I love and listen to my man I am fully present with my man, my man loves and listens to me, he is fully present with me.*"

As you say this and tune into it and really become it, it will start happening for you. Remember to let go and flow, not force it with desire. You must FEEL it, it has to come from the inner quantum subconscious fields, not from the outer mind.

Or, if you feel like your man is not honouring or loving you enough, then you might tune into the trauma that underlies this for a good half hour until you feel ti is cleared. Once the underlying trauma is cleared you will find the new mantra that your subconscious brings through, such as "*My man treats me like I am a precious being to be cherished and loved in all his spoken words and actions*". Then apply it to him "*I cherish my man like he is like a precious being to be cherished and loved in all my spoken words and actions*". And of course to yourself, "*I treat myself like I am a precious being to be cherished and loved in all my spoken words and actions*". You will find that the more you treat yourself like this, the more he will, too. This mirror will arise with your children too. But it has to come from within you. You must address the underlying subconscious inner trauma according the ways outlined in part one of this book.

You can work with the outer mind, using affirmations, but it is much better if they come form the subconscious once you have done the true inner trauma targeting. This way they come from a deep inner healing, and tackle your subconscious belief systems and conditioning programs. However you can also find mantras that resonate and if you do, the key with affirmations is that as you listen, take the light of them deep within to actually FEEL them within resetting your 'inner' energy fields and belief systems. But you have to take them to the inner.

So, for example, other mantras might include:
Men are good for me
Men are good to me
My man cherishes me
Men are gentle with me
(again, repeat the above also for yourself/all others)

"*As I love myself, other love me too and I love others. I am loveable, and i see that other people are, too! As I heal and love myself, I start to enjoy the person that I am and this is reflected in all of my relationships*"

Healing And Communication
Finding the time to communicate and tune in together, both during pregnancy and after the birth, is the foundation for your entire family.

If you are not in a relationship with the man who fathered your child, you need to be totally at ease with your feelings towards him, whether he is a former lover or a sperm donor. You need to work through any issues that you may have towards him and resolve them with forgiveness, acceptance and affirmation, as outlined in this book.

Once your relationship is healed and you are both empowered, you are ready to connect in a deeply loving space. Many of the most ecstatic births take place because birthing partners are able to connect and be present with one another in a fully empowered, deeply intimate, loving space.

Set up an intimate space for couple-meditation as a foundation to draw strength from and use conscious communication within it if you decide to talk in this space. Keep it focused and clear, begin and end with a candle. Loving support for your man means remembering to say thank you for all that he gives, to honour and respect him for all that he does for you. Use this meditation time for that. Sit in the relationship meditation space often, just be with each other or use some of the following meditations.

Try and continue this after the birth. It will be harder to find the time with a new born baby, but it is possible, anything is possible, and with mantra and manifestation you could find five minutes a day and half an hour a week to return to this intimate meditative partnership. You create the reality you walk into. This time is essential for the transition after birth and during the lack of intimate space many couples experience after having a baby. It will help keep you connected and loved as a man and woman, to feel honoured and united together. It is all about your intention, so do not force yourselves to do it.

This is the foundation for the family so find ways of creating it to be pleasurable, relaxed and easy.

Meditations for Loving Couples

Attracting Love Meditation
Your relationship with yourself is eternal. Your relationship with others, whoever they may be, is temporary.

Use this meditation to love yourself and enable others to love you with respect. You choose your destiny. Choose love by using this exercise. The Kissing Hands Yoga ritual is designed to bring in love and I have adapted it here to include mantras and visualisation. I met the father of my children the day after I did a loving forgiveness exercise on my own father, followed by inner male and inner female healing. If you do it for self love primarily, it will be mirrored in the relationships around you. Don't look for a man, look for yourself and the right man will come to you in the right way. Conditional love is the cause of relationship issues.

If you love yourself fully and meet all your needs, you won't be looking towards your partner to fill your needs.

Here's what to do: *Rest on your back with your hands by your side. Slowly bring your left hand to your mouth and kiss it whilst visualising receiving love. Then do the same with your right hand, now imagining giving love to yourself and to others.*

Imagine the following mantras and feel the meaning as if it were true for you right now whilst aligning the light behind the words to the inner. Noticing any blocks or icky feelings that might arise and face them. Bring them to resolution by addressing them with the technique in part one of this book.

I am loved and I love.
I am surrounded by love.
I attract love and I give love
Easily and well.
I deserve love.
I am truly loved.
I love myself and I love others.
Others love me.
I am truly loved by all.

Love is all around.
Likewise, I birth with love.
And birth in love.
Birth is love and love is birth.
I love.
I love.
Love.
So be it and so it is for the highest good of all concerned. Amen.

You can also repeat the Love Mantras given in chapter 2.

Loving Eyes Meditation

Sit still opposite your partner. Go to a deep place of relaxation. Now start to look into each other's eyes. You may like to focus on one eye. Just be aware of which eye, or if you "swap" eyes it does not matter. Just be with it. Don't judge it. Keep looking into the eyes. You are not looking for anything or for any special effects or experiences to occur. You are not analysing their pupils, or your emotions. Just keep looking and just being with the eyes. Look past thoughts, past judgements, past emotions if you can. Just be. Just be there, looking into the eyes of your birthing partner. Just sit like this for some time. Anything from 3 to 31 minutes. Just being. Just being. Together.

Male and Female Within Visualisation

Use in conjunction with the Full Power Self Meditation further on in this chapter. You can do this meditation alone or with your partner.

Close your eyes and go to your special garden. Relax. Breathe. Once you are relaxed, lie on your chair and just spend time being there.

Now ask for your Inner Female to enter the space.

See her enter. What is your first impression? Is she strong or weak? Tall or small? How does she hold herself? What emotions does she carry? What does she have to say to you and what do you have to say to her? Does she need healing?

Now ask your Inner Male to enter the space.

See him enter. Again, what is your first impression What does he have to say to you and what do you have to say to him? Does he need healing?

Now watch how they respond and interact with each other. Watch for some time and watch for messages.

Now ask for healing for your Inner Female.

Send her Christ light or Angelic Golden Light now. See her heal and shine and become her strong, true, powerful feminine self. See the feminine role as strong and powerful – not just the male within her. Now what does she have to do and how is she? How does your inner male respond to this?

Now ask for healing for your Inner Male.

Send him Christ Light or Angelic Golden Light now. See him heal and shine and become his strong true powerful male self. Now what does he have to do and how is he? How does your inner female respond to this?

Now see your inner male and female dance and interact with each other in a loving embrace, as the male and female embodiment of God. Two halves of one being. Simultaneously whole and powerful yet dancing in love and warmth.

How do they act, what do they do and say?

When you are ready, give them thanks and ask that they remain truly whole and powerful beings in this way.

Return to the room from your garden knowing that, for the highest good of all, your inner female and your inner male are now whole in their fullest power. So be it and so it is!

An Ode for Loving Union

What is loving union?
To be loved and cherished
And to love and cherish
To honour and respect
And to be honoured and respected
To be present with someone
And for someone to be present with me
To listen and empathise
To be listened to and empathised with
To share a journey of parenthood
To share a journey of loving and living
To have the time and space in ourselves to love each other
To recognise and support each other's dreams
To be on each other's side
To commit to resolving our shadows
as we look into our mirrors and recognise ourselves in the other
To create harmony with ourselves and our home and our children
To raise our children with light
To know we are thought of as right and worthy by the other
To feel truly within our own power and loved for it with the other
not with vows and promises of forever
but with the power of the now
Loving you is teaching me to love all others.
As we are one, so we are all one.
As I look at the Christ in you, so I see the Christ in me and in everyone.
We are all connected, we are not separate.
By loving you, I am able to reconnect with my own divine self – the I AM within.
To gently guide each other back to the path of truth when we have strayed
Not to personally take on all the other's struggles

To let you be who you are and to let you go your way even if it means doing things I don't want you to do or going places I don't want you to go

Knowing that true greatness, power and freedom in love is being able to do what you want to do not what you feel you should do

To create our dreams together

To walk the spiritual pathway of ascension together respecting and honouring our different languages

To accept and forgive our shadows and weaknesses and look instead at what we love about each other in the now

To work through our challenges with loving acceptance and forgiveness, alongside new skills such as conscious communication

To understand that whatever you do to another you do to yourself

To always kindly and tactfully speak our truth no matter how afraid we might be of the consequences

To manifest and affirm what we need from each other whilst being simultaneously in our fullness of power, needing nothing from each other but growing like two trees lending support, side by side.

I love this about you….

To be whole within so that I can love you clearly without any need

And as such whatever is right for you is right for me too.

Healing your Relationship with the Perineum Massage

From 36-40 weeks, you can commence the perineum massage using oils, perhaps almond oil.

This massage is an ideal time to bring loving forgiveness into your relationship and to create a beautiful intimate loving space for you both, with the ripples directly affecting your womb, baby and birth. Whilst doing the massage, you could ask your partner to speak words that you need to hear, like "I want to be with you and to love you", or to speak the mantras that you have written together or alone on your manifestation sheet. You can ask for healing or follow a visualisation in this book. If you want, you can look into each other's eyes whilst doing it. You may want to empower yourself by doing it alone, or else focus on the baby by looking away and turning within with your eyes closed. Play around with your intentions as you do it.

Be totally honest and feel any feelings that arise for you when your partner is in this space. If it does not feel right, don't do it. There are no 'should's, everything is right, use your intuition.

As well as using this massage time to heal your relationship in order to birth happily, **also use it as a time to imagine your cervix thinning from week 38** (as described in the healthy pregnant body meditation), and say words of release, mantras and thanks - for the highest good of all, so be it and so it is!

To do the massage

Use your fingers passively, as a focus to breathe out against. The stretching comes on the breath out. Insert two fingers into the vagina up to the first knuckle to start then later maybe the second. Press firmly against the back wall of the vagina towards the spine. That is all you do. At first you may feel like nothing is happening, but after doing it every day for several weeks you may notice the stretching, which comes from within the tissue itself. It will help your body to open up during the birth and to return to normal more quickly after the birth. It can also help avoid tearing.

To generally massage the area, use gentle strokes with no pressure to encourage blood flow. The vaginal tissues will be the most stretched so focus on these. You may like to do it in the bath or with a hot flannel.

Massage your nipples to promote healthy breast stimulation ready for feeding your baby. Nipple massage stimulates the hormonal production necessary for birthing. Do it with pelvis floor exercises and deep breathing.

Lovemaking in Pregnancy

During pregnancy, sex may be far from a woman's mind. Some people feel heightened desire, while for others, instead they crave loving embrace, sensuality and massage - maybe even orgasm, although this may be irrelevant. Whatever you truly feel is healthy and right for you, respect it.

After birth, I recommend taking your time to get back into penetrative intercourse. Your time is taken up wholly by giving your loving energy to your offspring and your yoni portal and has been through alot and needs sacred respect. To have to divert your energy to fulfil the sexual needs of your partner is neither balanced nor fair, unless you desire this also. However, your relationship also needs energy and loving. You can do this by opening up time for loving embrace and meditation and also by inviting your partner to love you without sex, and accepting his love and nourishment without guilt or the need to give sex in return, by instead bringing in Aphrodite and entering the temple of sensuality.

Many men feel left on the side and neglected after a baby arrives. So instead of neglecting him or giving him the sex he desires, instead invite sensual loving intimate time together.

You need time to be with yourself and to regain your energy as woman so that you can make love when you feel like it. Right away or after a year… it is irrelevant. We live in a time and culture that is too hung up on penetrative sex, that expects that a relationship will fail if penetrative sex does not happen frequently. Loving embrace is a far deeper connection for a couple.

If you have a balanced and loving relationship then your partner will nurture the woman who is devoting herself totally to the raising of his children. However, don't forget to devote some time to the relationship which is the family foundation as well. If you can't devote time to this then you need to tune into why this may be and try to empathise with a man who can easily feel left out.

Both fathering and mothering can be the loneliest job in the world sometimes. As you cradle and nurture your baby, either within the womb or without, you need your man to nourish, protect, worship and respect the mother-infant bond. If he feels jealous he needs to open up and face this with himself. If a man can be open and honest with himself and heal himself, he can then nourish his woman without expectation or sexual need. The man needs to be encouraged to find ways of positively and healthily supporting and giving to himself so that he can give to you and your coming baby: by hobbies, work, friends, walks, massages and treatments etc.

If a woman is nourished by a patient, loving man, then when the time is right for her she will return to sexual embrace in truly wholesome ways since he has not only honoured the mother-infant bond but also honoured her womanly needs whilst nourishing her to feel deeply loved.

2. By Connecting with you as an Empowered Woman

You might like to ask "What is an empowered woman?" Empowering yourself as a women allows the men in your life to be empowered too. What is a woman who is in the fullness of her power and of her woman-ness? Tune into your full power in the visualisation at the beginning of this chapter. Your power comes from you innermost self worth which you need to commit to every single day. Hand on heart hand on womb, being the divine fullness of all of you, complete self acceptance for all that you are.

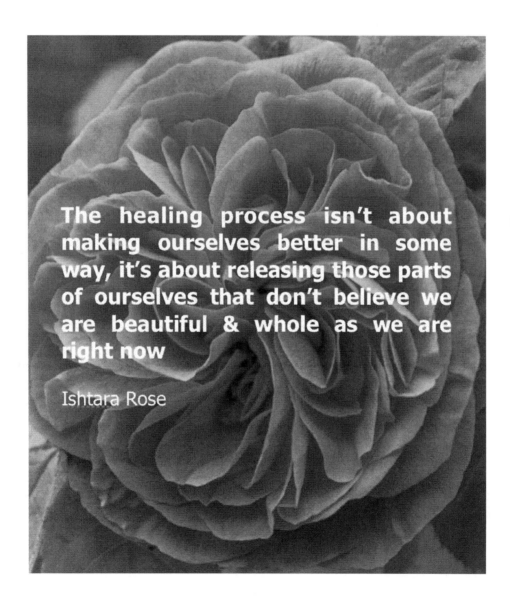

The healing process isn't about making ourselves better in some way, it's about releasing those parts of ourselves that don't believe we are beautiful & whole as we are right now

Ishtara Rose

We still live in patriarchal times with huge expectations and pressures on women. The expectations on women to deny their 'womanliness' are still huge: returning to work early, attitudes towards women who are full time mothers, likewise attitudes to women who return to work, terms such as "yummy mummy" for women who fulfil the ideal of being a sexy woman while juggling parenting with loving a man and fulfilling their career. Other examples we have discussed are the weight pressure - it is naturally right for some women to put on weight after birth when her milk comes in and she feels hungry for herself and her baby. Celebrate the full embodiment of being a whole woman, try not to deny it by feeling pressured to lose the weight so that you can look like teen air-brushed girls on magazine covers. Do what feels right for you and makes you feel good within (as opposed to feeding your ego to feel good). Keep on tuning in and following your own instincts.

The male aspect is the "doing" action, and the female aspect is the "being" (Sun and Moon, Yin and Yang). We each have yin and yang parts within us that equally make up the whole man or woman. The feminine aspect is the left side of the body, the energy of being-ness and inward-ness; the masculine aspect is the right hand side of the body, the energy of doing and outward-ness. Through the feminist movement, women began to emulate men as active and outward achievers, in order to have quality in the workplace and beyond, whereas some men who have become in tune with their feminine sides are judged as 'wet'. It is now time to balance the pendulum so that we can return to wholeness, where we hold male and female energy equally within us. A full woman is beyond expectations of achievement, or needing to look sexy or even having to look good. A full woman is in touch with her instincts. She is rooted. A true Earth Mother in all senses of the word. This is a whole new way of looking at it.

The history of woman in our cultural times is reflected in fashion. For example, trousers were invented at a time when women were trying to assert their power and equality by becoming like men, and mini skirts invented at a time when sexual liberation and experimentation mirrored the image of woman as a sex object. A strong woman in a long skirt is still a rare sight. (I am not advocating that you should only wear long skirts to be an empowered woman). When 'the pill' came in, many saw it as a form of liberation, but in some ways it was an attack on the divine womb, because not only of its side affects, but also because it enabled women to be liberal in their sexuality and give their sacred divine chalice away too easily, in the name of quality and liberation.

Women who remained in the sacred equality were called frigid and pious. Intuitive women are called irrational. Some people laugh at women for being 'brain-dead' in pregnancy and whilst feeding a baby after the birth. These are all derogatory beliefs that attack the divine feminine (and masculine because he needs his own female aspect and a woman who is fully embodied in her divine).

The 'brain-dead' state of being is natures way for enabling a woman to be in her divine aspect in her intuition and inner knowing. It happens also because hormones are released during feeding, and these hormones cut off the mind and make the mother feel dreamy. This happens for many reasons, one of which is that it enables you to be whole with your baby and to be completely in touch with your instincts, ready to birth and ready to meet your baby's needs. For example, you will catch the glass that falls well in advance, whereas a rational mind would not know it was about to fall. The release of these hormones and the subsequent feeling of being 'brain dead' also enable a new mother to juggle countless things at once (practical and mundane organisational aspects, alongside checking in with the well being of your baby and family in every aspect, often on no sleep). Isn't nature truly amazing? Let's celebrate it.

The ability to be totally in touch with your inner knowingness is summed up beautifully by Sophy Burnham in her book *A Book of Angels*:

"One day, when my babies were very small, I was working at my typewriter. We were living in Washington, D.C. at the time, not yet having moved to the Brooklyn apartment. One daughter was two, and the other, Molly, was only a few weeks old. I was working on the third floor of our little house in a little attic room. Down the corridor Molly lay asleep on the bed. Thought she was still too young to turn over (indeed had never tried to roll, though practised lifting her head), nevertheless I had caged her in between three pillows, just in case. She slept like a stone, flat out, as only dogs and babies can. In the other room I worked on an article, tap-tapping at my type writer (no computers yet), totally absorbed and concentrating on the work when –
Molly's falling off the bed, I thought, and in a flash was pounding down the hall to her room…where I caught her in midair.
Now, this is disturbing. Even if we accept thought transference or telepathy, how do we account for the fact that the baby could not have possibly known she was about to fall, much less transferred the thought to me? After all, she'd never rolled over before, never fallen, didn't know she was on a bed three feet in the air.
Moreover, I knew she was falling before the actual event. I had received information of a future act. Precognition, it is called."

I call this intuition, or inner knowing: the place we need to allow ourselves to be in, in order to birth in flow, to feed our babies with flow. The body knows this, which is why hormones are released to cut off the interfering mind. An empowered woman is in her full glory when she is pregnant and when she is what others may perceive as 'brain dead'. A woman's body knows what to do in birth - if it hasn't been repressed by thousands of years of patriarchal mind programming and filled with body altering chemicals.

Women were denied the political vote for many years, in part due to the belief that they were not in their rational mind during the menstrual cycle. However, if women are in a space of strong intuition at this time, perhaps this power was recognised on some level, and feared, which is why their vote was denied - something to think about. In Kundalini Yoga, women are believed to be able to have been given the blessing to be able to purify themselves monthly during their deep moon time, where as men have to perform yogic techniques to do so. Imagine what you can do when you are pregnant then. You can really use this time to deeply heal old wounds for your future generations (and for your ancestors).

Eckhart Tolle recognises that the female ability to birth and have monthly cycles (the womb-an), means that she is more in touch with creation - as well as her "pain-body" (ego).

"Generally speaking, it is easier for a woman to feel and be in her body, so she is naturally closer to Being and potentially closer to enlightenment than a man. This is why many ancient cultures instinctively chose female figures or analogies to represent or describe the formless and transcendental reality. It was often seen as a womb that gives birth to everything in creation and sustains and nourishes it during its life as form"
The power of NOW" by Eckhart Tolle

It is certainly true that in many workshops and courses on spirituality there are more women than men.

So in retaliation to hundreds of years of masculine domination, in order to be equal in the patriarchal scientific materialistic approach to living, women have taken on the masculine energy and denied the femininity within themselves. Feminism is thus another form of patriarchy and attack on the divine womb - it has denied the truly empowered Sacred Woman / Divine Mother.

Jessica Tomley, a top business woman said "I used to hate women until I had a baby. I never understood them". Once she had a baby, Jessica got in touch with her womanliness and decided to leave her job as a city worker to be a full time mother.

"Joanne was a lawyer with a strong background in feminism before motherhood struck and reports: The snag in the sharing of parental responsibility was that when the baby cried it was my breast, not my unsexist-very-willing-to-help partner's the baby wanted. All the equality I had negotiated in my relationship waned; my partner and I slipped shamelessly into gender roles: motherhood taunted the feminist in me. For the first time in my life, the feminist did not know what to say"

Buddhism for Mothers, Sarah Napthali

I also mistakenly believed that men and women were the same until I had a baby. I then realised how fundamentally different we are at many core levels, not just within our conditioning. The way my partner was within the home and in relation to our baby was so different to my own instinctual approaches, that I finally understood the differences between men and women. We are made differently. This Sun-Moon understanding helped me hugely when it came to certain resentments I felt towards my partner's behaviour and his opportunities as a man to be a parent and follow his own creative flow. For example, often women expect men to be like women and give moon energy but men are sun energy. Women want to talk and to be heard but men want to fix and move on. This is of course a generalisation, but it is important to understand this fundamental difference.

I began to understand the traditional roles that families played out, roles that I had never previously understood and thought were inhibiting or disrespected women, and for the first time understanding that these roles came about from the very essence of birthing babies. As such, I went from being a feminist believing in equality and having a career, to a belief in the Sacred Feminine / Divine Mother, in being a 'whole' mother who may (or may not) have a career as well. Yet she will need a man and a family and community support to do so, where as in the patriarchy, without that, the man can do both where as for her it is a fight and a struggle.

Women birth babies, who are then connected directly to our hearts via our breast. Women are one with their babies in ways that they simply cannot expect men to be. Joseph Chilton Pearce talks about the mother as the matrix for the child in his book *Magical Child*. He says that emotional security (thus intelligence, health and wellbeing of the child) depends upon the baby's security within the matrix, and the matrix's emotional happiness and connectedness to the baby in pregnancy, birth and the early years.

I do not advocate that a woman should relinquish herself and give herself totally to her children: it is essential that a woman retains a part of herself for herself, something which women practising holistic parenting may forget. Forgetting this essential truth can cause many repercussions for a woman and could ultimately be reflected by her children. Sadly this is often seen in spiritual and holistic communities where women are so child led that they have forgotten themselves.

Mothering and fathering are different and when you realise this, you can release your unrealistic expectations that men should be able to be mothers. This does not mean that men can't care for babies, change nappies etc., it just means that they have not birthed and fed babies, nor gone through the hormonal changes, and this influences the father-child connection in vital ways: they can care for their children but they are not interconnected. *Mothering and Fathering: the gender difference in child rearing*, by Thine Thevenin, covers this subject.

I am not advocating traditional relationships and stereotypical gender roles; traditional roles for man as protector and provider are also outdated. We both need to care for our children, but in ways that embrace our inherent gender differences rather than completely denying them. Indeed, positive choice parenting may mean in your family that the father is the key carer and the mother the key provider, and this can work well if the essential differences between male and female qualities are respected, understood and listened to. For example, attachment parenting can help a working mother reconnect after a day away, by carrying her baby in a sling as soon as she has returned from work, or co sleeping, to encourage as much close bonding as possible.

A happy mother is a mother who is happy within her relationship with herself, and with her husband; these relationships are your well for drawing strength. A baby is a gift of love and conceived from the love making act between man and woman. The relationships are, therefore, also the baby's foundation for being and essential for their wellbeing, as well as the foundation for the entire family. This often gets neglected during pregnancy, but for the baby and mother to thrive so too must these relationships. Note if the father is absent, this includes your feelings towards him affecting you well being and the family.

Whatever your situation, whether you are a single parent in a relationship with the father, sharing parenting with the father, the father is absent or there is no father in the family situation, you need to be nourished in your feelings about your love field. So you need to heal your feelings around your relationships not just to bring your child into the world peacefully but also in order to parent happily. This is not a question of berating yourself if you are in emotionally wounded situations, it is a question of self-healing and bringing love into your family situation, whatever it might be, as a secure energetic foundation for your baby. The mother can be nourished by a happy and loving resolution with the father, whatever their situation. Nourishment starts with loving support.

What does being a Divine Mother, a Sacred Mother, a Divine Feminine, mean to you?

What does having a womb mean to you?

How can you feel you womb as a sacred and divine chalice and how does feeling that change your approach to living and you self identity as a woman?

"On Earth, the Divine Feminine has been overlooked, misunderstood, misjudged, misrepresented and undermined...The time is now ripe for a Return of the Mother Principle... If we are embracing wholeness and Unity Consciousness on Earth, it is imperative that we familiarize ourselves with the "dual" nature of the Godhead. We have to

bring the heart into a gentle focus with the mind and balance the feminine and masculine within us…There are two permanent rays that penetrate the body of the earth. One is Masculine and the other is Feminine. The Masculine ray is considered gold and is anchored in the Himalayas. It is Lord Himalaya who is in charge there. The Feminine ray anchors in Lake Titicaca in South America. Its colour is pink. These two rays meet in the centre of the Earth and come into balance and fusion. The Feminine ray may for a time dominate in order to establish balance… Perhaps that is why there are more feminine beings opening up to Ascension and Spiritual Enlightenment on Earth than males. The majority of spiritual workshops lean more towards females than males in attendance. A Christ walks with a balanced Feminine and a balanced Masculine. There will be a Christ Race emerging on Planet Earth. But first the full integration of The Goddess."

Empowerment and Integration Through The Goddess by Rev. Wistancia Stone and Dr. Joshua David Stone

"Let the man worship woman as God, the Holy Mother, the Divine Shakti, the Mana, the Food of Life, the Sustainer of Being, Isis, Atarte, the Good Earth, Terrible Kali and Herself – All Of It. She is all of it. Let the woman worship man as God, the Son, the Sun, the Father, the Lite of her Life, the Creator, the Provider, as Jesus, as Ram, as Shiva, as Krishna, as all of them and Himself. Surrender and die to one another. Become One. The glorious Mystic Rose in the garden of the Heavenly Father. Permeate the Universe, fill it, become it for this is the union beyond duality."
Be Here Now by Ram Dass

I remember being told by a medicine woman in the Amazon "Do you know why they are really cutting down the rain forest? Because it is wet and dark and tangled and feminine."
Alberto Villoldo

3.   By Connecting with himself as a Healthy Empowered Man

In the birth space, you will pick up on whatever your birthing partner feels. If someone who is really tense gives you a massage, you will pick up on that vibe of tension. If you are tense, your baby is tense, as proved in *The Secret Life of the Unborn Child* by Dr Thomas Verny with John Kelly.

Therefore, it is essential that your birthing partner does whatever they need to do to be in a relaxed and positive space - in the pregnancy, in the birth and after the birth in parenting and supporting the mother. No pressure though! Remember this is within reason and with a balance for everyone getting their needs met with clear and loving respect for one another.

We have just discussed the need for a mother to be nourished by her man/partner, and he can best do this if he too is nourished and supported with his emotional needs also being met.

Help your partner to find positive and healthy support outside of the home. This may be with an alternative practitioner that he likes and chooses, or perhaps through a hobby of some kind. He needs a "birthing shaman" too and he may like to do some of the meditations in this book to find his helpers. If this is not his language, he can do it in other ways. Hopefully it will be someone or something that he can keep returning to after the baby is born to get some space for himself.

As well as understanding the differences between men and women, understanding the emotional abandonment that is the primary issue for expectant and new fathers can help you to stay empathetic towards your man after the birth. Many men experience a shock after a birth, a type of male postnatal depression, which can lead them to flee into a kind of absence to focus on providing for the family, whilst at the same time feeling threatened by the love and bonding that takes place between mother and baby. This can start in pregnancy. This first begin when a man gets very anxious and stressed about providing for his family. The man is also expected to support the family in a more hands on way, nappy changing as well as working, and this needs to be balanced in a way that is fair for all. Today it is often suggested that the man is being "unfair" by taking time out, but remember that he needs time too. However you balance the career – work – parenting aspects, remember that everyone must get their needs met.

After the birth, help take the load off your man by having meals provided for the family in the first few weeks or hiring a cleaner to do the housework. In that way, he can spend more time with you and the baby in a loving and sacred way. You both deserve help and since we no longer live in communities you must to create your own positive support so that you do not burn out.

According to Dr Scott Peck and Shannon Peck in their book *The Love You Deserve*, men in our culture are generally socialised to:

- Believe that they are protectors
- Believe that they are providers
- Believe that money is power
- Believe that they can control any situation
- Believe that women are inferior
- Believe in strength
- Believe in winning

This 'power' man (as opposed to 'empowered' man) is not trained for intimate love, for love that thrives on tenderness, sharing, giving and feeling. Like an empowered woman, an empowered man tunes into his heart and listens. Then he can listen to his woman and to her dreams as well as his. Use the meditation below as a guide for empowerment, as well as the Male and Female Within Visualisation above.

Full Power Self Meditation

This is another meditation (but different) to use to tune into your female and male and then to go beyond, into Source or Light. This version is written with a woman in mind, but can easily be altered for a man to do to tune into powerful man.

The symbol of the square and circle that I have chosen to use in this book came to me in meditation very clearly when I was pregnant just before birthing. Although the square and circle could be seen as male and female, the full circle seems to represent *oneness beyond gender.*

In birth it is important to connect with Divine oneness and not just one bit of it. So beyond all I have mentioned here about the empowered divine feminine and divine masculine, it needs to be clearly pointed out that man and woman are equal counterparts in one-ness in the heart.

Connect into the Divine mother, the female Goddess, do not deny her. Become her, luxuriate in her, birth from her. Then from here, reach and be connected with your oneness beyond gender. But always start with the divine womb portal and connect her to your heart.

One hand heart and one hand womb, feeling the two connected for some time with the breath.

Close your eyes, take deep breaths and just imagine yourself as a full and powerful woman... powerful from deep within, from God, not from ego. Tune into your full self and power as a woman. Tune into that part of you that is fully in power and loves you.
Really explore your feminine energy and what that means for you.

Then explore what it FEELS to be an empowered divine woman.
Really be with your power and breathe in more power if you need it. Breathe in your fullness of power as woman and feel full in your belly. Whole and full. Connected and full with Goddess in your belly. This is a place of self-honour and self-loving.
Write down any feelings that come to you as you do this.
You may create some mantras from this inner place of feeling, that are applicable to birthing in power.

Now tune into yourself as a reflection of the Divine Goddess and as the Divine Mother and connect with the mother energy. See the Divine Mother in front of you, tune into her and become her. It is time to embrace this energy and bring her back into your life. The mother is like the river: she nurtures and sustains all life that exists on, in and around her with love that is absolutely unconditional. Without her, life would not exist as she is everything. Her tides flow in and out and she nourishes all and whatever is done to her, she continues to be constantly giving. If we tune in and love the mother, she can flow and we can swim in clear waters. If you want to use the metaphor of your female self as a river, keep imagining that your waters are unpolluted (by negative thoughts) and keep light shining through you to make sure you are clear.

After you have tuned into yourself as a woman, you can then tune into your male self. What is man? What is a man's role and how does a power-full man hold himself? See the God in front of you and welcome him and honour him and his strength. Embrace the Masculine principle and welcome and love this energy of doing-ness and outward-ness.... Take your time...

Now you are a fully empowered person, your inner male and inner female are fully empowered and dance perfectly together. Affirm this for the highest good of all concerned. So be it and so it is!

Now you are in touch with your inner female and maleness, you will be able to tune into the part of you that is beyond gender, to be an empowered being. This I sometimes called the I AM energy. It is true power, filling the belly with pure Light.

Dwell in the Light for as long as you can.

When you return remember that this is who you are, and you may like to buy a crystal egg full of light to remind yourself of your inner source, and place it by the image of the Goddess that you have chosen for when you meditate and birth.

4.   By Preparing the Birth Space with You

Now that you have looked to your relationships and set up a beautiful intimate space, you can sit together and prepare the birth space by doing a Birth Rehearsal.

Once you have worked through this book to develop your birth plan, you can then discuss it with your partner and let him know what you want for yourself. Whilst the birth is important to both of you, his role is to support your needs as a birthing woman. Your responsibility to your baby is equal but it is your body and in this sense, birth is a woman's realm. Think about what you want as a woman first, then you can ask clearly, in your full power, for the support you want from him.

Once you have discussed the following you could do some birth rehearsals together. Birth rehearsals are outlined in the next chapter.

You may want to discuss the entire birth, all the possible outcomes and what you would choose in those situations, etc. You will want him to be absolutely familiar with your birth plan so that he can support it in every way necessary.

You may want to show him your birthing mantras and ask him to make his own, as well as creating some joint ones to use together.

You may need to rehearse massage techniques by learning them in a book, developing your own, or attending a class together.

You may want him to know where everything is: snacks, homeopathy kit (with clear, written instructions), etc.

You may want him to know a key word from your mantra exercises, such as "Golden Angel", which reminds you to relax and connect with the Divine Protector within if you are getting anxious.

You may want to have hand signals developed by you both to limit talking. Think about hand signals for "go away", "come here", "massage me", "get some snacks", "I would like a homeopathic remedy" and so on.

You may want a back-up plan in case things go "wrong" – you need to have a "what to do if?" conversation.

You may want clear instructions for how he is to deal with midwives and medical staff. Have a note and birth plan that you have signed, for him to refer to, so he has the power to make decisions on your behalf if intervention takes place.

You may want to have a sign for the door to back him up in case he forgets to say something or becomes anxious in a dramatic birth situation.

You could make up some cards or notes with headings for your man to refer to. Keep them simple, clear, easy, precise and short! There is an example of PROMPT CARDS at the end of the Birth Chapter.

He may probably need to be prepared for dealing with certain attitudes that medical staff may carry.

For example, when a back-up midwife arrived at our second home birth, it was in the middle of the night in mid-winter. In England, by law, two midwives should be present. However, we already had someone there who we liked and did not want anyone in our space that did not know how we were birthing. She came to the back door in an urgent way, waving a bright torch, ready to rush past Matthew to the emergency. He stopped her by standing across the doorway so she could not rush past and said words to the effect of *"Wait! This is our birth and we know what we are doing. We do not need or want you here, and Ishtara does not want you in the room with her. You need to wait downstairs. This is a Sacred birth. We are doing it in silence and in candle light. So please calm down, slow down and wait in the sitting room."* He thanked her for her understanding and presence. He needed to be very firm and direct with her as she was used to turning birth into to a dramatic emergency situation. Eventually she understood and kindly respected his wishes and we never saw her again, as she left immediately after the birth, having been downstairs drinking tea the whole time.

This is a time when the male and female aspects really come into their power. The woman is birthing, the man is holding the space. There is nothing sexist or 'gender-ist' about this! It is nature at its most divine.

You could print out some of the meditations in this book to refer to in emergency situations and to enable your birthing partner to be able to prompt you.

Finally, always remember this is your birth. Whilst this means everyone is there to support you and help you to create what you need and want, it also means that you need to be self-reliant. Even with the best intentions, your supporters may not be able to support you in the ways you desire. Do not give others your power and become a victim, be in control of your own needs. Others can support you but they cannot do it for you. At the end of the day, it is up to you to do it with the tools you have and the situations that arise. This also includes (especially includes) not giving power to your partner as a way to avoid taking responsibility for your own reality.

After you have done the manifestation programme, do the manifestation meditation together.

Tell each other your mantras and keep referring to them together to help with sacred parenting after the baby has been born.

For example, I remember reaching for my crying baby in the middle of the night in a tense way with hunched shoulders, and Matthew just put his hands on my shoulders in a very loving slow way saying *"slow down, slow down"* and the way he said it has stayed with me. Actually he didn't know that this was one of my mantras or that he was supporting my sacred parenting. But it was exactly what I needed to hear. Although we did many meditations together, I mostly did my manifestation daily practise alone and kept it from discussing too much with him so not to disperse the energy. This is mentioned in Part Three in the rules of the 40 day programme.

When discussing your birth plans together, remember *it is not what you say, but the way that you say it.*

Conscious Communication

Conscious communication means both listening to the otherand being listened to by the other. Listening means acknowledging and accepting what someone has said by repeating it back, empathising with the feelings and not trying to change it nor to talk about yourself or going into reaction. (See *Non Violent Communication* by Marshall B. Rosenberg)

Set the space as a meditation space to sit and talk with each other rather than trying to communicate at a busy time that could be interrupted.

For example. To listen to someone, you empathise with the person's feelings by mirroring their words and feelings:

Imagine yourself saying "I fell over in front of everyone this morning".

The person you were speaking to can choose to make any one the following responses:
"Oh well never mind" (this is dismissive)
"Silly you, are you ok?" (this is patronising)
"So, it doesn't matter" (this is again dismissive)
"Why did you do that?" (this is critical)
"Clumsy."(again this is critical)
"Oh dear, are you ok?" (this is fussing)

Now imagine empathy:
"Gosh that must have <u>felt </u>embarrassing"

The key is mirroring and validating the feeling.

So you listen to another by empathising and mirroring the feeling according to the statement, and then coming out of any reaction, and into stillness, you have the chance to express your feelings to someone who is open to listen.

Thus conscious communication is not just about listening to another, it also means talking to others clearly. We have to know how to talk consciously. State with clarity what you need and want from another and express what you truly mean by talking clearly from your heart. Try to eliminate waffle as well as noticing words and emotions that affect spoken words. For example, defensiveness, anger and shyness can prevent you from clearly stating what you want to say to the other person. Think about what you want to get out of a situation, rather than expressing hurt and talking about what you don't have. When you speak from your heart, if you say anything other than "I feel..." it usually becomes a comparison or a judgement from the place of ego.

When we are connected this all happens naturally without even attempting to do it. There is no effort and no attempt. But we must be connected in stillness within. When we are disconnected in our minds, then we revert into unconscious communication. Something we all do as humans when we are disconnected from the inner.

It is necessary to work on conscious communication in order to parent from your heart and really tune into your children and family. But that all starts with having space to connect within and find that point of centre and stillness.

What If My Birth Partner Cannot Support Me In the Ways that I would Like?

Your partner needs to understand intuitive and sacred birth and how it involves healing your inner fears, saying mantra and doing manifestation work alongside positive meditation and visualisations. He needs to support you on every step of the journey with an understanding of what you have taken on in your preparation for a happy birth. You may pick up on any tensions or unresolved feelings in the birth space. The energy and consciousness in the room affects the birth itself. If he has any unresolved emotions towards birth, his own or yours, and how you are approaching it, then it will be there in the space. So without ego projection and forcing ti is good to invite your partner needs to work on himself too in his own ways. The birth is important for you both, even though it is your body and, ultimately, your choice to birth in the way that is right for you.

Always ensure you are not being a victim and blaming your partner instead of becoming fully responsible for yourself. Your partner is free to be and do what is right for him at all times as long as it does not infringe upon your birthing peace.

"If the partner is not fully supportive of your commitment to ecstatic birth, although this may seem rather controversial, it is probably better that he is not at the birth. It has become a kind of orthodoxy now that the man has to be at the birth, and some men really, in their heart of hearts, don't want to be there, but they feel that they have to. It has to be done. If the partner is in so much fear about birth that he cannot support you in an ecstatic birth, it is more supportive for him to stay at home or go to the pub or whatever he might like to do. You can have a close woman friend or a relative or your breathwork practitioner, someone or ones who can really support you and be totally committed."
Valerie J Taylor, Midwife.

How would that make you feel?

If you resent his lack of support towards Sacred and intuitive birth, you need to deal with these feelings by practising meditations on acceptance and forgiveness and taking it to he steps in part one to target.

You need your partner to believe in you. If he cannot do that, don't see him as being wrong. Take responsibility, go to part one of this book, where do you create a situation where your partner does not believe in you. Own that. Step into your power. Target the trauma, Do what you must to tackle this and be empowered. Then find the birth support you need and want from someone who does believe in you and may also be able to help him to do so, perhaps a Doula or a friend.

Refer to the discussion on relationship healing above and use the manifestation plan and mantras to heal the trauma, as well as to attract the emotions you would like in your life. People say that you cannot change a man. However you can empower yourself and changes may be mirrored in the relationships around you.

Examples might be - Be subtle. So you might like to initiate a candle lit space and take the lead with massage and mantra instead of saying "let's do a meditation on Thursday". You could ask him to say certain things to you or say things to him without using the term 'mantra' if that challenges him etc.

Being in your power in pregnancy means being in your fullness as a divine womb (woman) in a loving and harmonious space. If your partner cannot love or respect you, you need to make changes within the relationship. If you are in an abusive relationship you must alter it or leave it – whatever is necessary. If you are in an abusive situation you must remove your child from it. Take action within but also without. Do whatever makes you feel in harmony for your birth. Keep on referring to the manifestation chart with your mantras and rituals. You deserve abundance and love.

Acceptance and forgiveness towards your partner is also very important. Acceptance and forgiveness does not excuse abuse, but it opens a pathway to being empowered to let the abusive other go. It has to be found within by healing and targeting the root trauma to come into your power, with support. This is who he is and how he is now. That must be accepted rather than trying to change him. So allowing him to be who he is does not excuse abuse, but enables you to let him go and let him be. The feelings "you should..." express expectations that are the basis of victim consciousness. They really say to the absuive other "I will accept you as you are but just moan about it". If you truly come out of trauma dependancy and into deep empowerment from tackling the inner subconscious and doing the inner healing, you can easily walk away knowing you are whole and do not depend on him for anything. A man does not have to be anything but himself. It is you who decides to be with him and whether to have him at your birth or not. You need to accept him for who he is and get on and do what you need to do. You have a choice. Rise in your power and get on with things. Find support elsewhere, maybe in an alternative practitioner. Allowing him to be who he is will enable you to be who you are.

Remember to make any mantras that you make about him applicable for yourself as well. I.e. your man is not present with you. Feel into the feeling of "my man is present with me" and then "I am present with myself" and use part one to target the trauma or root belief causing the feeling or situation of his absence.

As discussed in the tension releasing chapter, once you have worked on something, let it go. Do not dwell on what does not work, but on what does. Tune into pain only in the space you have created to do so (with an energy healer for example or at home in a designated space with a journal) but then let it go and tune into the positive state, do not carry it around outside of that allocated time. Then you can be present in the now with your pregnancy and baby. Try to be conscious: don't expect him to take the lead with this, be in your power and take the lead for yourself. If conversations are getting heated, you are in your power to deal with them as you would like. The more you empower yourself and communicate consciously, the more you allow others to do so as well. Lead by example.

First always come out of mind and reaction, go into the inner space, as outlined in Part one.

7 - Clear Birth

Silence!

Sacred Birth in Progress!

Please limit intervention.
We prefer to have silence in this room.

We have chosen to have a Sacred Birth using Intuitive Birthing Techniques taken from the Manifest Sacred Birth Programme.

The Manifest Sacred Birth Programme is based upon keeping the birthing mother in an uninterrupted trance state in tune with her intuition.

Please help us to maintain this by treating this birthing space as a sacred place and by being as quiet as possible.

Thank you for your support.

Reminder of the Basics of Intuitive and Sacred Birth

You are looking to birth from a trance state.

Anything that interrupts this trance may cause tension or slow the birth down. This is the main cause of complications in birth, which can be resolved either through the use of meditation techniques to regain the trance state or through the use of medical intervention methods. You must always follow your intuition for the right resolution for you and your baby.

Sacred not scared. Connected within the heart womb, not in mind.

The primary cause of pain and trauma in birth comes from the tension and anxiety. This may be caused by your environment, but whatever it is, it affects your internal emotions and your response to your situation. Therefore, you need to be in the most relaxed place you can for the birth itself, and be able to respond in a relaxed way to whatever occurs.

The secondary cause of pain and trauma comes from external unnatural environments, toxic people, loud talking, bright lights, as well as drugs and medicines that are invasive, unnatural and have side effects. Knowledge of natural healing methods, including mantra as well as herbs, can give you alternatives and coping mechanisms if invasive pharmaceutical medicines and other techniques are suggested/employed.

You can immediately go into a vibration of love and peace at any time by focusing on your chosen Goddess image which you can place on you birthing altar with your mantras. See the Divine Mother meditation in the Clear Spirit Chapter.

It is essential to reconsider ancient knowledge about the unique female power of reproduction & birth if we are to change the current trend towards unnecessary and painful intervention during birth. Ironically, it is often only in so-called civilised cultures that birthing women experience pain. In many tribal cultures, birth and menstrual cycles are considered gifts that are both enjoyable and empowering (a blessing, not a curse).

There are four stages in a Sacred Birth -

Stage One	Surges are established/The Great Opening Up
Stage Two	Birthing the baby
Stage Three	Birthing the placenta and being with your baby
Stage Four	Welcoming your baby for the first few weeks and beyond

Relaxation

The importance of being relaxed during birth cannot be emphasised strongly enough. Birth is an intimate dance with yourself, your body and your baby. Whatever, and whomever, makes you tense should be removed from the birthing space immediately. Whatever, and whomever, makes you feel at ease is your birthing right. Birth where ever you feel most relaxed according to your intuition. This may be at home, a birth centre, or even a hospital. You know what is right for you.

The intimate birth dance could also be described as being in a trance state. This trance state is the deeply relaxed state that you are looking to achieve. During birth, take your time to really luxuriate in the sacred vibes of your femininity.

Ensure that anything you do or take in the birth space does not interrupt the birth flow or take you out of the birth dance (trance).

Pain Free Birth Comes From Staying In the "OM"

The first doctor to realise that tension in the birth space causes trauma which leads to the need for intervention was Dr Grantly Dick-Read, in 1913. He discovered that relaxation gave rise to positive and pain-free births and that the women who were relaxed in birth were those who were not lying on their backs (which inhibits the backbone and causes pain – a position invented in Victorian times for the doctor's ease) and those who were not in hospitals. He was the first to realise that many wealthy women birthed in pain in hospitals, whereas tribal and peasant women often birthed with ease at home. He made important links between pain and fear which introduced new ideas about birthing practices in Western society. His story is outlined in his book *Childbirth without Fear.*

"Mothers who are afraid tend to secrete hormones that delay or inhibit birth…those who are not terrified are more likely to secrete in abundance the hormones that make labour and birth easier and less painful – sometimes even pleasurable".
Ina May Gaskin.

Ina May Gaskin discusses one woman who experienced orgasmic birth and afterwards said *"I just went ahead and enjoyed myself!"*

Do you remember the monkey that I mentioned earlier? Indeed, taking a closer look at other *wild* birthing mammals shows that they often hide away in safe, hidden places to birth in private. They do not have other animals observing and examining them and, furthermore, will not birth if they are in unfamiliar environments or with a distracting noise or watchful human: if they cannot find a safe and private space to birth quietly, alone, then they will try to hold off until they can. Like wild animals, women unconsciously inhibit birth if it feels unsafe. In the UK, Midwives are required by law to observe the birthing woman.

During my second birth, I became aware that some of the slowing down and pain that I experienced upon opening was due to:

1. Going into my busy mind and my worries regarding my other child
2. Not connecting with my baby
3. Tension about my relationship expectations being let down
4. Feeling invaded and self consciousness about a watching midwife (who was also a neighbour, which highlighted the feeling of being watched by the village).

The first midwife had entered the room to observe. My partner and I had specifically requested privacy but at this point my partner was in another room with my toddler. The midwife was observing in a respectful way, she was a yoga student and sat by the candle cross-legged, smiling peacefully, but watching. I came out of my bodily presence and became aware of myself. My partner said that the sounds I was making changed and became much more self-conscious. Things slowed down and I immediately thought "why is this happening? What is happening? What shall I do about it?" Despite all my learnings, I started talking to the midwife to discuss it and try and resolve it! I totally forgot to reconnect within! Luckily my partner came into the room and asked her to leave.

At the time, I was quite happy for her to stay and cross with him for interfering! But left alone I was able to reconnect within, leaving behind my self-consciousness and getting back into trance by meditating. From that time alone, reconnecting, I was also able to reconnect with my baby within as a be-ing, not as a boy (whatever implications that had for me). Then as I reconnected to my baby, I had an urge to release in the bathroom. As I ran there, I saw in another room that my daughter was playing happily, watched over by my partner.

So suddenly all four issues were neatly resolved in one moment, simply by reconnecting within. The neatness and synchronicity of this was also due to the mantra, manifestation and visualisation work that I had been practicing to heal myself whilst working with spirit guides and was able to put into practise in the birth space when left alone.

Like many other women I have spoken with, the slowing down that occurred could have taken a different path and led me into a traumatic experience with a need for intervention. Luckily, my partner noticed and requested that the midwife leave and then I was able to put my meditative techniques into practise. If I had reconnected within and felt that I needed intervention, I would have needed to remain in a calm meditative space as much as possible throughout whatever intervention was needed. It is possible to have a Sacred birth even in an invasive medical environment if you are able to reconnect within. You must listen to your intuition to follow what is needed for you and your child, and to do this you must always connect within, into the birth dance.

Why did I slow down?

Well first, it has to be said here that there is always a slowing down in between the stages. This is part of natures rhythms. So we must embrace the pause and know how to remain connected within the pause.

But I did not remain connected in the pause, first because I forgot that the pause is natural and second because I went into mind. This was when I was being watched. I was thinking as opposed to being in the dance. I was tense because of personal issues that I had been working on resolving in the pregnancy - concern about my toddler, tense about my relationship. I was in a parent space, rather than an intimate space. My partner had been working hard – we were not in a love making space and I was resentful. I was worried about coping with two babies. There were many factors which had created a tension which I worked on releasing. Furthermore, I felt very alone in creating a home birth – alone in my approach to birthing and parenting in alternative ways without a supportive system in place. . I was juggling many things but I used the methods in this book to acknowledge and resolve them.

I want to highlight here how, considering all this, the manifestation work **still** paid off and I had the birth that I wanted. The pain shifted into sensation by focused chanting and protection invocation to be in a safe sacred space, held by my partner.

Furthermore, after both of my births I learnt from the baffled NHS midwife that the placenta was disrupted in some way and that it was an *unexplained miracle* that all had been well for mother and baby - twice! Also there had been a major artery that had been in the way in the first birth, and it was a miracle it hadn't been ruptured when a midwife tried to break the waters (with no success).

It is very apparent that pain is created by tension. It really is that simple. If you are in a Garden of Eden, supported by people you love, at ease in your dream, you will have a pain-free, happy, easy birth.

Yet few of us are in that space and that is why we have to work at creating that space in the ways outlined in this book. Do what you need to do to be connected and relaxed. Do not berate yourself if you do not reach your pain free, home birth aims, we have after all thousands of years of patriarchal ancestral conditioning to work though. babies also have their own karma. Having said that, miracles do happen, healing can happen in the blink of an eye when all in ripe, and many women have birthed pain free and in beautiful flow naturally at home through these techniques which re align the inner frequency and energetic patterning.

The Ark was Made by Amateurs, the Titanic by Experts

Currently, many hospitals and medical centres do not support creating harmonious birth via relaxation and creation of trance states but aim to get babies out by any method necessary in invasive patriarchal imposing ways. This includes methods that are forced, destructive, dangerous and emotionally disturbing with long-term ill effects. These methods inhibit the trance state which is the very thing needed to birth well. Birthing in hospitals is often violent, intrusive, painful and disempowering.

Many women do not realise this, they bury a negative experience and put it behind them, left with mixed emotions towards hospitals staff ranging from gratitude for their devoted 'help' in clearing up the side affects of the invasive methods that they believe 'saved' and 'helped' them, to anger at their invasion, or a deep inner niggle feeling of disempowerment without understanding why. This is because most women are exhausted after birthing and just so grateful for any help and then left with a new born baby to deal with and the elated feelings of that. The invasive methods can be violent and overt or they can be more subtle and psychological, and if a woman is not in touch with her sacred womb needs she will have no idea how abusive the invasive birthing methods have been.

According to the National Childbirth Trust in the UK, studies have shown that problems are much more likely to result during a hospital birth, such as babies born with a lower Apgar score, interventions such as episiotomy, drugs for pain, drips to speed up labour, infections after birth, difficulty in feeding and so forth. This is also because fo what is called the wheel fo intervention in pharmaceutical approaches - once on measure is taken, it leads to a side affect that another measure needs to be taken for and so the chain begins.

Home births, on the other hand, enable women to feel more in control and more relaxed. Most people thinking about a home birth are concerned with something going wrong, but transfer to hospital is fairly quick wherever you are. Things 'go wrong' if you disconnect and become tense. The biggest cause of transfer to hospital found in home births in these studies was due to the slowing down of "labour" resulting from a pressure and an anxiety towards birth.

If however, you feel that birthing in a Birth Centre will encourage relaxation for you, then you need to go with that. Some people feel that they cannot relax in their homes and need to be in a Birth Centre of some sort with a support system around them. Unfortunately, it can be a struggle to find a natural birthing centre, and you may have to go to another country or find ways of setting it up at home. If you do prefer to go ahead at a midwifery unit or hospital, do your ceremony and ask the universe to ensure that the right staff and people are present to make it a harmonious situation.

Although I do not wish to dwell on the negativity and violence in hospitals, it is important if you choose an empowered birth to understand some of the history of birth in this culture, to empower yourself with knowledge about birth. This will help you decide where and how you want to birth. If you decide you want to birth in a hospital environment, and if tension arises, you will be more prepared to deal with it as you will be aware of the pros and cons.

Everyone I have met who has had a difficult birth has experienced tension of some kind. Sadly, the primary creators for tension are the primary birth carers themselves. Out of the many women I have spoken to about their birth tension, most stated that they felt self-conscious and un-relaxed in the presence and observation of midwives and doctors. There seemed to be a recurrent factor for all of these women: not only did they feel tense, this made them shift into a thinking/analytical space, turning away from their bodies and instincts.

Hospitals and medical staff are not interested in the soul, they do not see the person and they do not see birth as sacred. However caring they seem, they have to follow legal guidelines that do not respect sacred birth. Furthermore, they cannot support intimate trance dance. Hospital environments are places that are coming from the 'mind' practising medicine that is based on the philosophy of Louis Pasteur. The environments are unnatural and opposite to the quiet sacred temple cave that all birthing animals in nature will seek out. Bright lights, observation, loud talking, medical drugs that create side effects and a lot of fear-based decisions. None of the factors in a hospital environment are supportive of a sacred, intimate and quiet birth.

Would you make love in the presence of a stranger taking notes?
To be overt, can you defecate in front of a stranger?

These are good questions to ask because birthing is a very intimate process. It is difficult for most human beings to create relaxed, intimate, trance-inducing vibes under bright lights and observation.

Maintaining Privacy and Stillness
So with this in mind, it is also good to consider how anything that changes your environment (perhaps getting in a car or even just talking) can break the birth trance.

When Tanya's surges slowed down she started walking around whilst talking about all sorts of things to her midwife. Her birth ended up in a painful induction because the midwife convinced her to go to hospital and she entered into a chain of intervention. In retrospect she says she wishes she had been silent and still and not gone into her mind. She says she knew she did not need to go and felt talked into it. She says she felt belittled and invaded, and in that space she lost her confidence to follow her needs. feels grateful to the medical staff for their help and support and at the same time angry for their interference and inability to support her emotional needs and not being able to support her to go into the pause at home. She felt it was not necessary to go to hospital, she gave her power away and she had a painful induction. Yet she had a lovely baby girl who was born healthy and they were both looked after there for a few days. So she felt conflicted in her blame and anger to them and or herself for not being 'able' to maintain her space, as well as appreciative for their support. This contradictory emotion can be likened to the feeling a child has for an abusive parent – love and gratitude alongside anger and hurt. Tanya has worked on her worth, she has healed her resentment, and she also no longer sees her birth as a failure simply because it did not go how she wished, and she understands the growth that came from all that she uncovered in her healing work.

Now interestingly Ava was also going for a home birth like Tanya, and she also ended up having induction in hospital when things slowed down and yet she just knew she had to have that, and that DID actually save her and her baby and she feels a genuine gratitude towards those who helped get her to the birth centre fast and in a gentle way to support her birth wishes to maintain a sacred space even in the circumstances. She met staff who respected her birth plan and aims, despite no longer being at home.

So here are two stories which both ended up in induction, with two very different end results. All spending on how empowered the woman feels to follow her own gut intuition and inner knowing.

Once things have slowed down and a birthing woman feels self-conscious or disempowered, like Tanya did, inner tension arises and the medical professionals often advise hospitalisation and induction or caesarean. A birthing shaman would instead advise techniques to aid relaxation so the birthing woman can return to her power and instinct and know what she needs to do, or simply leave her alone for a short while to go back into her power and birth trance, in her own ways.

Question everything that you are told and keep tuning into your intuition. For example, if your waters have flowed or if medical staff have examined you, you may be told that induction is necessary within 12 hours due to risk of infection, even though this risk of infection is minor. This creates pressure to get on and birth quickly from a place of fear, even though many people naturally and happily birth many days after their waters released. This is a prime example of a situation that causes intervention. Remember that after intervention takes place, there can be a "chain of intervention". One thing can lead to another, i.e. examination leads to induction, one drug has a side effect so another is given to counter act this. Yet with the awareness in tact, if you know you need to go to hospital then you do have the power to make it good and not feel like a failure (if you wanted a home birth) just as Ava did.

It is all about the inner knowing.

The focus on maintaining privacy and stillness in the birth space to be in that space fo inner knowing, is essential. Start feeling more about how you can do this and how you could turn it around and come back to you power, if you ended up in a place you did not want to be in or being convinced to go somewhere you did not feel like you needed to. So feel into ways how you could reconnect within if things slowed down. Also remembering that there is always a 'slow down' between the different birthing stages which is part of a normal and natural birthing process.

The Birth Rehearsal

Please do not start this until you reach the forty day birth manifestation programme, then start to do it as often as it feels right to do so.

This rehearsal will enable you and your partner to be empowered in birth by being prepared for all circumstances. If you have rehearsed this both alone and together, then you can have more confidence to find it easier to surrender to birth, with limited talking and interruptive communication. In turn, you can tune into YOUR intuition constantly – and so be in the right place at the right time for you and your baby.

This is your chance to go through each stage of the birth and imagine, visualise and affirm how it will be for you in both essence and form. You and your baby communicate telepathically so this is also a rehearsal for your baby and your body.

This is your chance to think about what you really want in birth and to practise it. This is also your chance to amalgamate all that you have learnt in this book and to make it your own, and then to communicate it clearly to your birth partner, ready to rehearse together.

For your birth rehearsal, I strongly suggest that you refer to the following meditations and exercises in this book:

◦ Your Mantra Sheet. These mantras make up a big part of your rehearsal; they are the essence of your birth and incorporate your clear mind and clear emotions

◦ The clear emotions and clear mind meditations to help with quick and easy fear release

◦ The healthy pregnant body visualisation as well as other healthy body meditations in this book such as Body Surrender

◦ The clear spirit meditations, to remind you of easy ways to connect within

◦ The clear connection meditations, to develop such things as partner sign language

◦ The three stages of birth, using as much detail as you want.

◦ The Natural Birth Pain Management Chart, Birth Anxiety Chart and Birth Centering Charts; including such things as birth mantras, visualisations and massage techniques.

Example of a Birth Rehearsal

The surge begins

Mother: *I signal to my partner that a surge has begun and then get into the position that feels right. I then signal to my partner to massage me, rub me, or leave me alone.*

I refer to my visualisations and breathe with them, using my affirmations as a mantra and words that make me feel relaxed…every sensation tells me that my cervix is opening beautifully…

Partner: *I stop what I am doing to be silently present with her, either in the room or not, whichever is needed. I observe her body for signs, such as any tension. If she is opening and responding well to my presence and touch then I join her in her relaxed breathing perhaps with light touch massage. I stay relaxed n myself, so she will tune into this relaxed state within me. I am birthing along with her too, so I remind myself about the need for me to breathe and relax.*

I refer to the prompt card to help remind me to support what she wants and I continue to use positive language to help her to open such as YES and I BELIEVE IN YOU.

If I notice tension in her, I use words to remind her to relax , saying her affirmations and words that she likes to hear to cue her to relax, as previously discussed - things such as "well done, relax, loose jaw, relax into the surge, your cervix is now opening, surrender to it…". I just keep on responding to her signals with sensitivity, loving kindness and belief in her, whilst protecting her space to birth as she wishes.

I place my hands on her and invoke the angels by saying 3 times "I ask to be a clear channel for light and love and healing, may this mother and child birth in light" and fill my hands with gold and white light.

The Surge has ended

Mother:
I remain in my heart and my body and try not to go into a talking space. If something is bothering me I go within and chant the appropriate words or go to my garden and talk to my baby and my heart. I summon the angelic beings to guide me. I go to the toilet if I need to, otherwise I roll my hips and stretch and prepare for the next sensations by relaxing and trancing out with positive opening. I keep on with my affirmations and visualisations at all times even whilst the sensations have stopped.

I refer to my prompt card for a key word to repeat and a visualisation, if I come out of my trance and need help getting back in.

Partner:
I have already lit the candles, and now give her some arnica and rescue remedy and honey in water, in a subtle way so as not to interrupt her trance, if it feels ok to be in the room. I help her change positions, go to the loo, or share and listen to her concerns with my heart and hugs.

If she wants to reconnect with me, I try and initiate it with eye contact rather than words.

*If she goes into a head space and starts to talk, I bring her back into her body by...
(removing the midwife/leaving the room myself/massaging her back etc.)*

*If she has fear or anxiety, I help her to return to a relaxed, inward, silent trance state, by
saying her affirmations whilst massaging reassuringly. If something is bothering her, I let
her express it so that she can reconcile it within. My presence reassures and aids but does
not invade or intrude. I protect her space from others when appropriate. I am silent at all
times but say affirmations or play soft music that she loves if needed. I trust my own
intuition to know what is needed and respond to it, without having to ask her.*

*I repeat soft encouraging words gently like a mantra such as "your cervix is opening now"
and "breathe, relax, well done"*

The Birth Reminder Card

Write out your reminders clearly for yourself or your partner to refer to in the birthing
space. Keep it very, very short - five things may even be too much. You could even just
have two words on this card. It ideally will be an amalgamation of everything that you have
learnt in this book.

It might include:

5 key mantras
5 key phrases
5 key words
5 visualisation signals – names of guides or words to remind you of a relaxing
visualisation/experience from the exercises in this book

Other things you could add to the prompt card:
Massage techniques you like
Music you like
Homeopathy and oils that are essential for you
Reminders of birthing methods
Relaxation techniques that work for you such as a yoga pose or loose jaw and 'breathe',
'eye contact'
Reminders of words and mantras, no talking, signals, positive language
Reminders of things that make you feel turned in to God, in a trance, and full of LOVE in a
state of utter surrender, peace and happiness, relaxing and riding with the flows within

The Birth Plan

The birth plan is a simple document which allows you to record your birth wishes for all to
read. It will protect your space and enable your partner to implement any wishes you may
have in order to retain the sacred birth essence should you end up in a hospital
environment or operating theatre.

The birth plan is an affirmation in itself. Therefore, whilst you plan for any eventualities, you
write it assuming that the birth will take place as detailed in the plan. It is your clear birth
intention. Refer to your affirmations and keep it simple and clear. Once you have written it,

remember to keep in the flow and let go, following things that "hum" for you, even if they are not on your plan.

You could keep this document in a file with a list of phone numbers of friends and family and the intuitive birthing note for the Midwife in this book (Supporting Intuitive Birth – A note for those present). Keep these alongside your natural remedies and perhaps a note for the door for after the birth which thanks visitors but requests privacy.

The following is an example to guide you in making your own personal plan.

It is fairly long as it includes lots of things for you to consider for yourself. Choose the key things that call you. The main plan comprises the birthing form. You might like to add key notes about the birthing essence as well.

Our Birth Plan

We are choosing to have an intuitive and sacred home birth using intuitive birthing techniques that we have rehearsed and learnt in the intuitive birthing program.

As a result, we respectfully ask that the following be honoured in both the essence and form of our birth space:

Essence.
   1.   Safe space which is quiet, gentle, nurturing and calm.
Anyone who enters the space to do so in a calm, un-rushed fashion, in silence. We do not want busy, rushed energy around us. We would like to be undisturbed unless we ask for assistance.

   2.   Birthing from intuition within.
Christa wants to listen to her animal instincts and follow what she needs to in every given moment. As a result, no-one can tell her what she needs to do, and the following plan could change. It is imperative that Christa can be honoured and respected as a person to make her own decisions and thus be in her power as a birthing mother.

Form.
During Birth please respect our wishes for:
○ limited intervention (includes limited paperwork), for us to be left alone to birth using techniques learnt.
○ silence - no talking.

- my other child's presence to be respected with loving kindness. If <u>we decide</u> that her presence is not conducive for everyone's highest good then we will take action with back up plans in place.
- time and space to be left undisturbed
- freedom to move and experiment with natural positions
- to use natural techniques if an issue arises, and given privacy to do so.
- use of positive language (give example – sensation instead of pain).
- no monitoring and no examinations unless requested.
- to make my own decisions
- no coaching on descent of baby and delivery to take its natural course. To birth from yogic breathing as opposed to pushing. Nursing staff presence to be minimal and to be supportive of natural birth.
- to create a sacred space with candles, music etc.

After Birth:

- retain silence and encourage the birthing mother to do so
- the first words are those of the parents, no one announces gender, etc.
- privacy – time for us to be left alone with our baby.
- only for us to touch our baby and have intimate contact.
- skin to skin contact and immediate suckling.
- cord is not cut until permission granted when it is no longer pulsating, and then cut by ourselves.
- partner to stay with mother and baby, no separation of any family members at any time unless requested by mother.
- vegetarian and wheat free diet.
- time alone with my other children.
- no injections or supplements of any kind unless permission granted.
- to keep the placenta.
- the vernix to be absorbed and not cleaned away.

If a medical situation should arise, we will retain the essence of intuitive sacred birthing by:

○ minimum intervention

○ clear explanations and clear time to decide (birthing mother has the right to claim her birth space as her own, to be empowered within it by making all decisions at all times with clear information given and entrusts this decision making to her partner should it be necessary)

○ time to be alone and not rush, to create a sense of calm whatever the situation

○ birth through silence and breathing.

○ a sense of sacred calm and silence in the operating theatre with partner present at all times and bonding for mother and baby to take place in privacy afterwards.

I ask that minimum medical intervention is given and take full responsibility for my natural birth. It is my desire to refrain from the use of artificial drugs at all times unless requested.

Signed_____

We thank you for your attention and respect.

Information for Carers - Supporting Sacred Birth

This birthing couple have been learning specific intuitive birthing techniques as part of the Intuitive Birthing Programme to manifest Sacred Birth

What is a Sacred and Intuitive Birth?
Intuitive birth means remaining relaxed and in a meditative, private space in order to birth both sacredly and happily from the mother's intuition.

If a birthing mother is in a relaxed trance state, she can access her intuition easily, trusting that her body knows how to birth.

This is an ancient technique used in primitive cultures and currently growing in popularity since recent studies have proved its success.

The mother will appreciate being helped to remain in a relaxed "trance –like" state with encouragement and reminders from those people present in her birthing space.

How Can I Support This Birth?

This birthing couple have learnt specific techniques as outlined in the Intuitive Birthing Programme. As a Midwife, you can support this couple to achieve the birth that they have been working towards by:

Tuning into *your* intuition and acting in the birth space from a place of sacredness and being present with *your* higher self.

Encouraging them and reminding them about the birth they are hoping for.

Honouring their wishes.

Respecting their privacy by keeping a distance. The birthing mother must not feel observed or self-conscious at any time.

Letting them have power over all decisions within their birth space.

Encouraging the mother to remain in a meditative trance space.

Using positive language such as sensation instead of pain, birth instead of labour or surge instead of contraction.

No talking in the birth space - limited talking to the partner and no talking to the mother – she must not go into her head space.

Respecting sacred space such as dimmed lights, relaxing music.

Allowing the mother to be as active or inactive as she chooses.

Having faith in the mother's intuitive ability to birth her baby herself.

Being open and supporting them from your heart whilst trusting your own intuition at all times too.

Please be aware that, like other natural birthing techniques, Sacred birthing mothers using intuitive birthing techniques will be so empowered and relaxed in the birth space that sometimes it may actually not seem as if the birth is fully established when it is.

Dealing with issues during the different stages of the birth itself

You understand clearly now how you can use your mantras for anything and everything, if they are birthed through the inner quantum field within your subconscious.

So you can also bring any special circumstance in pregnancy to the quantum inner space to clear out any blocks and re align to a more aligned flow. Such as, breech babies, overdue babies, anaemia, or in birth surges slowing down, meconium, baby getting stuck), or after birth jaundice, tears in the perineum, mastitis, and into parenting colic, night waking, behavioural issues... these are all events that are reflections of energy frequency, everythgiq starts in the energy and emotions within the subconscious or quantum fields.

Your children live in your energy field and whilst they are their own people with their own karma, they also act out whatever is going on for you emotionally. All healing commences with the 2 aspects - first feeling into the feminine (the water in the cup and emotions behind things) and then also looking at the masculine (the container or cup that holds, the action without). Your instincts are you compass: only you know the truth for your family, other knows best.

"God gave us faces, we make our own expressions."

Remember, everything has ongoing effects and it is you (not the medical people nor the author of this book) who live with the lifelong implications and impacts of your decisions. You have to be sure of what you decide and take full responsibility for your decisions, you take always have a choice and it is always you that makes that choice.

When thinking about birthing issues, you might like to ask:

What would I do if this happened?

What would my partner do?

How have I/we coped with issues previously?

How can I apply the methods in this book to prevent it from happening before or in the birth itself?

Stage One - The Great Opening Up

Opening Yourself Up Wide

To open yourself up wide, you need to feel very safe.
The power comes from the feeling and belief in being safe.
With this power you can say YES to your body with every surge.

In stage one, when surges are established, your body is opening up ready to birth. This can take anything from one hour to four or more days. An average hospital birth is around eight hours, sacred births differ as the mother is more relaxed and may be having surges without knowing it, although this is still often denied by mainstream midwives. If you are relaxed, **your cervix easily opens up to the right size required for your baby and for your body**, thus it is a myth that birthing a large baby is painful.

There are three layers of muscle in the uterus: the outer layer has vertical muscles that align with your baby and the inner layer has horizontal circular muscles around your baby. The thickest part of the circular muscles is around the bottom of the cervix and if these relax and thin your baby can emerge more easily. During birth, the outer layer draws up and around your uterus at the top, which in turn pushes your baby downwards whilst causing the circular muscles to open. If you are relaxed, this thinning and opening stage is easier as the muscles work in harmony together as they are designed to do.

Dealing with Pain In Stage One

Pain is experienced when one is somehow not at ease with the opening and thinning sensations. Women can have orgasms when birthing, it does not have to be painful and the sensation can be transformed into deepening ones of joy. However we have years of programming to undo and so do not berate yourself if you do experience pain during this process. The following suggestions will enable you to relax the muscles and enjoy the sensations more, to help you dive into the pain and allow it, to make it sacred, rather than to tighten in fear and the scared, thus enabling you to travel through it. We are looking to turn the scared into the sacred but remember not to berate yourself if you have pain, as said, there are thousands of years of conditioning here.

"If our pain is perceived as an unwelcome curse, we will gladly have it taken away. When we do, we cannot fathom what our body is doing as her voice is silenced"
GeorGina Kelly, Midwife.

"Why did I not know that birth is the pinnacle where women discover the courage to become mothers?"
The Red Tent by Anita Diamant.

Birth is a big event but one that is totally natural. How much you can open depends on how relaxed you are and how your body creates the necessary hormones. You will release oxytocin and endorphins if you are relaxed.

Natural Pain Management in Stage One

Do whatever enables you to go into trance state. You may find some of these suggestions very helpful or you may find them counterproductive and they may actually interfere with the rhythm and intimate dance you are looking to achieve and create more tension. Just keep following your instincts. They might be that you need medical attention and that you need to step away from your dream birth plan. Your instincts are always right. If you end up in an exceptionally painful situation then do not be afraid of bypassing induction completely and asking for an epidural or caesarean. You can protect the sacred essence of your birth and use your birthing knowledge to ensure minimum trauma for you both whatever the situation.

If a situation arises that needs help, remember to explore the natural ways first. Ask yourself "what am I tense about and what will help?" For instance, nipple stimulation can get things moving if the surges have slowed down.

Think about coping with sensation rather than removing it, since if you are focusing on it going away, it could create more pressure.

Support
Remember to be with people who can support you to birth by tuning in. If they can't, ask them to leave. If you feel invaded, ask people to leave you alone. Your birth partner needs to be on top of this to hold you space for you so you can be left to go into the trance.

Acceptance and Surrender

Remember, surrender is not giving up your power to accept what other people are telling you to do. Surrender is about saying YES to your Self. Think about how easy you find it to surrender in everyday life and start practising this art now.

"I was so in my head during my first birth, trying to think my way out of this painful dilemma. I squirmed and tried to push away the pain. The pain only intensified. Although I was committed to natural childbirth, after twenty four hours of labour I was ready to just cut the baby out. But I knew I didn't really want that. My midwife in her good wisdom sent over a friend (Mary) who was very jolly and round. Her babies practically fell out of her. Mary positioned herself in the bed next to me and said "It's a bit like surfing. Let's ride these contractions." She taught me how to let go and surf with the force of nature. And then it became bliss. It occurred to me that a lot of (my) pain was caused by resistance to surrender. I was fighting it, trying to get away from the pain. I was judgmental to myself, wondering why I couldn't do it right…"
Birthing from Within, Pam England

Emotions

Release any hang-ups with mantra and fear release. Emotional support from a loved one is essential. Check up on your emotions towards your partner, do you feel loving and open? Voice any concerns if you need to do so. Allow yourself to receive all the love and support around you. Open to receive support. This is a difficult task for many women and especially difficult to ask for.

Relaxed jaw

The first step to relaxation is to wobble your jaw, with or without sound.

Sound

When I was tense, I transformed pain back into surges by chanting.

- Sound. Tune into the part of your body where you feel the sensation and give it a sound. Start with "aaahhhhh" or a tongue wobble, or even an "aye aye aye aye aye".
- Mantras. Find a mantra to repeat: a single spiritual word like "OM" or your mantras from Part One - "I surrender my birth to God", or chanting the names of the Masters and Beings of Light.
- Ina May Gaskin says *"true words spoken can sometimes relax pelvic muscles by* discharging emotions *that effectively block further progress in labour"*. So say whatever you need to!
- Remember, the power of words in the birth space cannot be underestimated. Tell your body to relax. Your body does what it is told. Remember positive language. Saying "YES" will help your body to open and saying NO will tense it up. Say YES to every surge. And talk to your baby.

Colour

The colour that you pick in the birth may surprise you. Find a colour and imagine it encircled around the part of you that is tense. Breathe it in and out and imagine it healing you. Feel it inside that part of you.

Visualisation

You will now be practising the daily visualisations that were suggested in the healthy pregnant body meditation, such as baby positioning and cervix thinning, alongside the perineum massage described in the previous chapter. You could also imagine more bodily functions happening, such as hormones being released, muscles moving, etc. If you want to do this, find out about what happens during birth and imagine it happening. Beware of birth language if you do this. For example, there are hypnosis recordings that are quite specific, but these can use negative birth language such as words like "contraction". You could also imagine -

- ○ a waterfall cleansing away the pain
- ○ the sunlight healing it
- ○ a rose opening to enable your cervix to open wide
- ○ a balloon drifting off
- ○ blue lights opening up your cervix
- ○ a spiral that you twirl around
- ○ waves rolling onto the shore

Breath

KEEP ON BREATHING! Stopping breathing creates tension.
Use breath to enhance visualisations, colours and chants.

Breathing exercises for staying calm:

1. Breathe IN relaxation/colour/light/water and breathe OUT tension and pain.
2. Breathe IN light and as you breathe OUT imagine it flowing all over and into your body. Do not focus on the pain at all.
3. Practise yogic breathing in between surges by focusing on breathing slowly: breathe in for 4 counts and out of the nose for longer, maybe 6–8 counts, drawing the breath over the back of the throat.
4. Use confidence boosting breath - inhale through the nose then exhale powerfully through the mouth making sounds like "shhhhhh". Repeat until calm.
5. During surges themselves, you could breathe in deeper and for longer, maybe even 15 counts or more, and see the breath going deep down to your baby and vagina. Breathe through each surge alongside your visualisations.

Holographic Breathing

Holographic Breathing is a natural, self-healing system which is helpful in birth. In this type of breathing, the breath is through the nose and there is a specific movement of the mouth: on the in-breath the jaw opens, and on the out-breath it closes. This movement is contained by the lips being closed, and the tongue being on the roof of the mouth. These different motions complement each other. They also create a natural dynamic that allows the face to gently open, and close with the breath. In effect the face starts to breath. This is then reflected through the cranium and body, including the pelvis which also starts to breathe. There are several seminars relating to the pelvis in Holographic Breathing. In the first of these, participants learn how all the different bones of the pelvis breathe and move. In this process the pelvis becomes a very fluid structure: it is designed to give birth. In the experience of birth this ability is very helpful, allowing the pelvis to breathe with the baby.

One of the advantages of this type of breathing is that many women say it takes away about 60 % of the pain of labour or changes it to something more orgasmic.

Homeopathy

Purchase a kit, see a specialist or make up your own homeopathic birthing kit. Even if you don't use it, having it there might ensure peace of mind, which in turn could make the difference between a good or a tense birth.

These can be used as long *as they don't interfere with the rhythm and the intimate dance.* You may find that to take pills/snacks/drinks could bring you out of the birth trance.

Rescue remedy	Take every 15 mins or so (this is a Bach Flower Remedy. You can use flower remedies in conjunction with homeopathy. Whilst choosing them you can do so randomly, with the use of a reference book, guided by instinct or see a Practitioner).
Aconite 200c	For anxiety and fear. Give if the mother fears she will die or something will go wrong or if the birth feels too fast.
Arnica 200c	Give afterwards for healing. Can take every half hour whilst birthing to ease swelling. Helps if tired and weary during birth with surges that are too feeble to be effective. First choice for haemorrhage. Mother says she is fine but clearly is not, may be feeling sore and bruised and keeps needing to change position (especially back).
Carbo veg 200c	Weakness, especially after loss of fluids and blood.
Caulophyllum	Useful for false sensations or to soften the cervix from 38 weeks. Use only with direction from a qualified Homeopath. Also helps expel placenta.
Chamomile 200c	Useful if mother can't bear sensations and is getting very angry.
China 30c	For post birth fluid loss and post birth exhaustion.
Cimifunga 30c	For false surging sensations.
Gelsemium 200c	For if baby feels as though it is going up rather than going down.
Hamamelis 30c	For piles after birthing.
Ipecacuanlia 30c	For nausea, haemorrhage.
Kali phos	For exhaustion and shakes post birth (often happens – shamans call it the incarnation dance or rattle).
Kali carb 200c	Good if sensation stays in back.
Luprum met 30c	Use for leg cramps.
Nat mur 200c	Give a single dose for back pain.
Platina 200c	Good if external parts are very sensitive. Can help relieve piles.
Phosohorus 200c	For profuse post birth bleeding.
Pulsatilla 200c	If mother is very weepy and feels she cannot go on, or if surges slow down.
Secale 30c	Increased post birth bleeding.
Sepia 200c	For Needlelike bearing down sensations. Take for after birth piles.
Sabina	Give a single dose to expel placenta

Crystals

Birth moss agate, jade, moonstone, opal, peridot, blue-green smithsonite.

Massage

Massage classes for partners to learn specific techniques for the birth are on offer in various places. Only use massage if it makes you feel relaxed and enables you to be with yourself – again, you may find that it could bring you out of the trance rather than enhance it.

Acupressure points

There are many pain relieving points in the body to access in childbirth, as well as ones that promote easier transition or opening of the cervix. A few pain relieving points include -

1.   Hand points: if you grip a comb in your hand so that the teeth of the comb touch the points in the creases of the hand where the fingers join the palm, endorphins will be released into the body.

2.   Yongquan kid-1: this point lies in the depression found in the top one third of the sole of the foot.

3.   Hegu L.I.-4: found between the first and second metacarpal bones (of the thumb and first finger). It lies at the point where the thumb is brought to rest against the index finger.

Reiki, (and different types of energy healing)

Learn this and do it yourself or have someone you feel relaxed with doing it for you in the birth, or invoke the rays as described in the Clear Spirit Chapter.

Herbs

See shock tea and juices in section below. Take Siberian ginseng for strength.

Water Birth

Immersion in water will ease any strong sensations. The benefits of using water in birth include:

Feeling in control and satisfied

Relaxation, soothing and comforting sensations, like having a warm bath.

Being more relaxed means less painful and shorter births

Easier to create quiet space and thus less intervention and more privacy

Studies have shown less chance of tears and less need for episiotomy (due to being relaxed)

Fewer babies need to be admitted to special care units

There are seemingly no disadvantages and no health concerns have been found.

Dealing with Anxiety in Stage One

"Whilst birthing my first child, I spent over four hours in my second stage, with very little progress. The energy dissipated, my rushes finally rushed off, and I didn't feel like I was any longer in labour. I had lost the urge to push – which was the phase I had been dreading without properly addressing, all through my pregnancy. I made token efforts to push – but felt like my baby was stuck. I said "no" to the impulse to push, so it vanished. Fortunately I was at home with my partner and my closest friend, a midwife. They both gave me the time and the freedom to work out my fear. I ultimately became conscious of my need to confront my anxiety, and trust myself to push my baby out. I chose to whisper an intense 'Yes', the 'great Yes' in my heart, and instantly the rushes returned with power. Tilda was then born very quickly after this, into the hands of her father."

Georgina Kelly, Midwife.

Shock tea for birthing
This recipe is taken from "Holistic Herbal for Mother and Baby" by Kitty Champion. Mix 2 tablespoons of apple cider vinegar, an eighth of a cup of honey or maple syrup and a full tablespoon of cayenne powder. You can sip through a straw throughout birth and it will stop the onset of any shock as well as warm the mother's body by increasing the circulation, raising blood sugar to provide energy and prevent danger of haemorrhage. Grape and apple juice and ginger tea can stimulate the organs, so these can also help but don't take at the actual time of birth due to risk of haemorrhage.

Birth Calming Checklist for an Anxious Mother

Add your own to the following list:

- Do whatever you can to say YES to birthing your baby.
- Mantra-mantra-mantra and visualise-visualise-visualise whilst letting-go-to God!
- Tuning in and connecting to baby, body, self and spirit guides.
- Focus on a meditation in this book and keep on repeating it
- Listen to your body. Remember: listening… keep listening to your emotions and internal needs and follow the energy so that you can differentiate between fear and intuition.
- Is there anything you need to release? What are you anxious about? Do you need to ask anyone to leave? Nothing is silly, even the smallest of things is greatly important if it is interfering with your birth.
- Follow your instincts – they might be entirely different to what you think.
- Remember Ina May's Monkey, surrender and hand birthing over to your body and your baby and your God(s).
- Stay present with yourself and your baby, avoid conversation and be as alone as possible.
- You can birth from your safe space, keep returning to being there and listening for messages from guides.
- Do whatever you want to be at ease.
- Create sacred space.
- Commune with spirit guides and Ancient Midwives.
- Talk to your baby's spirit.
- Put up protection with white light.
- Ask those present to be as quiet as possible.
- You may like to have a sign made up to place on the door requesting quiet.
- Telling your body what to do in the birth space works!

Birth Calming Checklist for an Emergency Situation

- Follow the Ten Step Fear Release Action Plan and find you own unique mantra from your subconscious.
- Follow the protection exercise and return to your safe space.
- Remember to tune into the opposite state of calm - visualise it and become it with affirmation whilst letting go.
- Deep breathing as described above in the painful birth suggestions.
- Pray and call upon all birthing women, everywhere, all who have ever birthed, to

come and help you right now!

◦ Eliminate whatever is bothering you, whether it's the "relaxing" music that you are listening to or the presence of someone you do not want there.

◦ Don't be tempted to talk and analyse.

◦ Learn to differentiate between fear and intuition (see chapter on clear emotions).

◦ Exercises – throw or beat things to release pent up emotion.

◦ Hot bath and a meditation or visualisation on your ipod.

◦ Massage with gentle music and oils, it might take 30 minutes to calm you down but loving touch often works.

◦ Hypnobirthing – rehearsed birthing cues and touches

◦ Make sounds or repeat mantras, either one of your own or a general one such as "I surrender to God", "All is well in the eyes of god", "I release birthing to my body and to my baby". Or repeat a mantra such as "om nama shivaya" or simply "it's ok, it's ok, it's ok". Create time, eliminate pressure.

◦ Read this book or a spiritual text, refer to your birth manifestation sheet and affirmations.

◦ Light a candle.

◦ Look at a beautiful picture or view, or focus on the Divine Mother image on your birthing altar.

◦ Use loving forgiveness and acceptance from the "we are all one" section of this book.

◦ Remember you have the right to refuse any treatment or procedure even if it is routine at the place you birth in.

"Overdue" Baby

I put this in inverted commas since in my perspective, there is no such thing as "overdue". The term means only that you have passed a given due date which is based on an 'approximation'. Once more, you can only follow your own intuition on this: whilst some argue that being five days past your due date is life threatening, others think that inducing a baby before they are ready to arrive is also life threatening and unnecessarily traumatic. Only you know if you are too late or if something is wrong or right.

Only 5% of babies come on their due date. Anything up to three weeks past your due date can be normal.

First babies are usually overdue. However, if your baby is very late then there could be something you are anxious about. Research shows that babies born in war zones are usually overdue. Or it might be that it is simply not the right time for your baby yet. You need to relax and eliminate whatever is bothering you - in your home, relationship or birth space.

Our first baby was three weeks overdue. Interestingly, I knew that I had to birth at three weeks and gave myself that deadline. When my baby was born and I had a placenta that was starting to decay, I saw that my intuition was right. Intuitively I knew that I could not induce (I later discovered that having my membranes ruptured would have been life threatening for both myself and my baby) but nor could I wait more than three weeks. So I had to resolve any issues to bring on the birth before three weeks, without feeling pressured! In this situation, I went into birth immediately once I had released my anger towards my neighbour and their dog that was always barking near my bedroom window (invasion issues).and once I had accepted that induction would be ok. I decided that in this situation, a caesarean was completely natural since everything is natural and of the earth and that I would be ok and did not need to fight that anymore. Once that anxiety was healed, I was able to birth with ease.

What issues do you need to clear up?

Use the visualisations in this book to tune in.

Just let go and don't worry, don't research, talk, think, etc. **Try not to *make* things happen but *let* things happen**. (The ironic key formula to manifestation). If you feel you must do something, you could -

- RELAX
- Do a ritual and find some specific mantras from Part One
- Ask and talk to your body
- Release fear using the exercises in this book
- Find a herbal remedy
- Take castor oil (the author holds no responsibility for this - do your research)
- Have penetrative sex (prostaglandins in semen can soften the cervix)
- Have an orgasm - orgasm releases oxytocin and may encourage movement
- Eat sperm and pineapple (!)
- Exercise
- Have a membrane sweep (do this in a very gentle way whilst talking to your cervix)
- Check you are feeling loving and open towards your partner, good about your body and in tune with yourself
- Have some acupuncture, reflexology, shiatsu...

Medical induction sets off a cascade of intervention and you may be drawn into the world of drips, electronic monitoring, epidurals, and all the other trappings of a medically complicated birth. If, after two weeks past your due date you are being pressured for induction you could decide to compromise by having regular monitoring... use your intuition!

Breach Baby

If your baby is breech, you may want to see if you can turn your baby into a natural birthing position that is right for you both.

Remember, your baby and your body know what position they need to be in, not the text books. You may feel that it is right for the baby to be in the position that they are in, whatever that may be. This may be a challenging statement for some people.

If you still think it is not 'right' then tune into the emotional and mental causes and perhaps into your own birth. If you try to turn your baby using the following methods and these do not work, you may decide to birth her/him naturally in that position (I have heard tales of many healthy, natural, magical breech births) or you may decide you want intervention. If you go down the road of intervention you can still keep the birth Sacred and take all the necessary steps to keep it so. You always have a choice.

1. Tune in, connect and release any shadows:

◦ Go within: talk to your baby and to your heart. Go to your garden in meditation or try automatic writing, and ask questions such as: why have you attracted this situation? What is emotionally upside down in your birth? Is your baby happy birthing like this or does your baby want to tell you something? If your baby needs to turn for birth and does not want to birth like this, ask how can we do this? Maybe your baby needs to be in this position, maybe there is nothing wrong with it, maybe you don't have all the information and this needs to happen for some reason.

◦ Use the manifestation plan and fear release action plan to correct things. Find help through alternative therapies.

2. Be in the Light. Now you have tuned in and resolved any issues, you can let go and focus purely on positive images and words:

◦ Use visualisation and mantra. As outlined in the healthy pregnant body meditation, affirm and visualise your baby in the right position constantly until you know it is all ok, and can affirm it 100% knowingly. KNOW YOUR BABY IS IN THE RIGHT POSITION FOR YOU BOTH. Most books, for ease of drawing and seeing the baby in the womb, show the baby the "wrong" way around: they depict a baby so that you can see it's face in the drawing. In fact, you need to imagine your baby with its head facing towards your bottom. Imagine and know that your baby is facing this "right" way around. Affirm and trust that your baby is in the optimal birth position for a natural, easy and healthy birth – he/she knows what that is.

◦ Do some exercises whilst affirming and visualising, to encourage optimal foetal position. These include using upright and forward leaning postures to allow space for baby to turn, kneeling on all fours, sitting with knees higher than hips, sitting upright on chair leaning forward slightly, leaning forwards whilst standing and swaying your hips, kneeling on floor over large beanbag to read/watch television, sitting leaning forward over the back of a chair in front of you, swimming with abdomen forward. Avoid lying on your back, long car journeys, legs crossed... However, if you are going to follow specific advice of "dos and don'ts", always use your intuition first. Your own body's truth could differ from the advice given.

Cesarean Birth

Many caesareans are for breech babies who have been booked into the operating theatre before their due date. These operations are not only unnecessary could create long term effects for the mother and baby. Caesarean sections may result in loss of power from not having had a vaginal birth, underweight babies, trauma, difficulties with bonding and more.

Think about these issues and *if you feel intuitively that this is the only way for you and your baby*, think about how you can turn it into an empowering and positive sacred birth, because you can create a cesarean Birth to be empowering and sacred. But please only proceed with this if you are sure it is the way forward for you and not a fear based decision or one based on convenience.

Ensure that you are clear about your decision to have a caesarean and remember after hearing the information that it is your right to do as you feel despite the opinions you are given (for example, to go home when it suits you). Question everything you are told. Things you might like to ask/think about might include:

- Do I want the surgeon to talk about what is happening?
- Do I want to watch the birth with a mirror?
- Do I want to cut the cord?
- How many people will be present and do I want them there?
- Having the procedure explained clearly.
- Being clear about why I need it.
- Being clear about whether I can wait until my baby is full term and if not, why not?
- Understanding the exact process and how I could deal with it - i.e. do I need to be catheterised and when?
- Being aware of the side effects of anaesthetics and deciding how to deal with this.
- Knowing how long you need to be there for.

If you end up unexpectedly in theatre having a caesarean birth, think about how you could keep your birth sacred and empowering. Examples might include -

- Use the fear release and anxiety charts in this book to clear and/or heal any reasons why you feel that cannot have the birth you want.
- Use affirmations and chant them out loud or silently in your head as the operation takes place.
- Talk to your baby about what is happening and why.
- Keep your partner with you at all times to protect the birth essence, and be clear in what sort of circumstances he might leave if he has to.
- Set the space to remain sacred: ask for use of dimmed lights when the baby is born if possible.
- Invoke angelic beings.
- Keep the placenta.
- Ask for quiet.
- Bring down healing energy to wrap around you and your baby.
- Wrap baby in a blanket that has your smell immediately after birth.
- Aim for immediate suckling on breast.
- Play music.
- Ask for an atmosphere of calm to encourage better bonding.
- Have your hands free to touch the baby.
- Not have the baby's gender announced.
- Cuddle your baby immediately as you are stitched up, while affirming and visualising protection for you both

Do not be disappointed if some of your expectations and hopes can't be met, let the experience unfold in its own way. Let go once you have requested, but at the same time do not be afraid to remind someone of your requests if it is important to you.

Stage Two - Birthing the Baby!

In stage two the baby emerges. If you have done the perineum massage this stage will probably be no longer than twenty minutes. There are differing theories on the overbearing urge that many women experience to 'push' their baby out. Some people say that you should try and breathe past this urge as you may not be ready. In my births I could never defy nature's urge to release, and tried to go with it using breaths that enabled my baby to emerge slowly and gently.

Try to use the word "release" instead of "push" - you do not want to push your baby into the world but instead release and ease him or her out using breathing. When you feel the urge to push, drop into deep 'breathing down'. Just keep breathing down. There are various breathing techniques that you can practise, or you can just follow your intuition instead and go with whatever feels right at the time. The aim is to do it slowly and with ease.

It is a beautiful experience to place your hand down and touch your baby's head as it emerges. This is a feeling that will stay with you forever. Keep relaxing until the next wave comes to birth the rest of your baby's body. Go with the waves, your body is doing it. All you need to do is relax and stay in the flow, visualising a flowing, emerging baby.

You can sing your baby out with clear focus. Keep absolutely intent and focused on what you are doing with visualisation, sound, talking and breath. Do not let anything or anyone take you away from the focus.

Stage Three - Birthing the Placenta and Being with your Baby

Protect the space.

This is the final stage of birthing and is an extremely sacred space that enables the bonding process and sets the energetic precedent for parenting and child wellbeing.

Immediately after the baby emerges, it may seem as if the job is done. Lights may be put on and the sacredness of the birth may be forgotten. This is the point at which you need to remember to focus on maintaining the sacredness you want. Keep hold of quiet now, more than at any other time, as this is the baby's first encounter with the world. It is a deeply sacred time. Mother and baby should never be separated, lights should be dimmed, no one should talk and the atmosphere should remain like this for hours or even days.

Keep the atmosphere silent and sacred. You could be so overwhelmed by the birth that you could start talking and giving the baby to someone else to hold whilst you wash or put the lights back on, etc. If you do lose your centre and thus interrupt the sacred space, have your partner ready to gently maintain this space for you. You will appreciate this later on. This is your baby's first taste of the outside world of form and the first few days are ones to be protected from unwanted visitors and kept sacred.

This is the time when Doctors and Midwives are keen to come and make sure everything is alright - turning on lights, shining torches in baby's eyes, talking and questioning, clearing up the "mess" and mopping the floor, injecting baby with artificial substances, taking the baby away to give the mother a rest and so on. Beware!

Whether or not you decide to go along with these interventions, you have to be very strong in your power to keep the space sacred.

The Cord and the After-Birth

My Placenta releases and comes out naturally and easily, gently and smoothly.

The birth is not over.
Maintain the space.
Stay within.

Some medical practitioners believe that as soon as your baby comes out into the world, the cord should be cut. This was standard practice in the UK for many years.

It is essential, however, not to cut the cord until (at the very least) it stops pulsating. I recommend keeping it attached long after it has stopped pulsating. Some people keep it attached for days or weeks until it drops off of its own accord. Think about who you want to cut the cord if you want to cut it – yourself, partner, child or another.

The vernix (white substance on baby's skin) should not be washed off as this is an extremely beneficial healing ointment. If anything, it could be licked off.

Some people keep the placenta for the welcome ritual or eat it as it is incredibly nutritious and healing. It could also be slowly dried in an oven on a very low setting, then ground into a powder and used as medicine to feed the mother's energy in the first few weeks. There are many placenta encapsulation specialists in the UK who could do this for you if you did not want to do it yourself.

The time between the baby coming out of the mother's body and the placenta coming out is the most sacred time in your child's life. If your placenta is taking its time to come out, let it takes its time. This is obviously needed. Relax into it. If you feel you want to help nudge things on gently then use nipple stimulation or nurse your baby. This will create a powerful uterine contraction. Or take a tea: drink raspberry tea with honey, and/or dong quai. Try to accept and let things be and do not rush, you have all the time in the world. If needs be, tune in and see if there are any issues that need resolution.

Some people like to get their baby sucking on the nipple as soon as he/she comes out of the womb and onto their chest as this helps the placenta to come out and is beautiful for the baby. Other people say that their baby does not want to feed much immediately or even for the first few days as he/she is slowly incarnating and just taking his/her time. All babies are different. Follow your instincts and do not be alarmed.

Stage Four - Welcoming your Baby for the First Few Weeks and Beyond

Stage Four begins immediately after Stage Three and is the beginning of Intuitive and Sacred Parenting.

At the end of Stage Three you need to protect your space from people coming to help out by washing and clearing away. The time you spend in a pool of blood with your baby will be the most grounded you will ever feel in your life. Dwell in it and luxuriate in it, do not rush to tidy it up. Take your time. When my partner tidied up the birthing space before I was ready, I felt like I had lost something sacred. It felt very invasive and as if the birth had not happened or had been swept away as a dirty event (he thought he was doing the right thing!).

I recommend being in that space and maintaining it for days, well into stage four if possible, and not letting any outsiders (including family) into it. They are the surest things to burst your birthing bubble, no matter who they are or how much you love them. If you must see them, see them in another space. This is intimate space. This is private birth space to be protected at all costs, for you and your baby to incarnate into. If people do not understand this and take it personally, that is their problem - do not take it on board as yours. Your place is to be with your baby. You owe that to your baby and yourself. This is self love and self respect. You can welcome others as soon as the time is right, to share your joy with them. But it must be when the time is right in the right space.

The most common complaint that mothers and families in this culture make after birth seems to be that their beautiful baby bliss bubble was burst instantly when other people came into the space. Someone else's presence in a room changes the atmosphere dramatically. It is within your rights to ask your family to give you the time you need to welcome your baby. If they are upset by this then they are not supporting you or your baby and are interested only in meeting their own needs. On the other hand, you do not want to cut yourself off from the world and from other people. Think beforehand about what you would like as you will probably be overwhelmed by calls and visitors and may not realise that this is problematic at the time.

I had this in mind in my first pregnancy and asked my family for space before and after the birth. They did not understand and even thought I might be depressed! They kept pressing to visit with excuses to bring things around. I had to fight to maintain my space in the last few weeks. After the birth, I was so elated that I invited my mother over immediately. This meant that my father also came, as well as my in-laws later in the afternoon, to be fair to everyone. I thought it was fine at the time but realised later that this was the one thing I regretted, that it had burst the special birthing bubble too quickly, especially since my mother in law wore strong perfume that lingered on my baby for the first week. My rush back into the world after our first birth (to mother and baby yoga and for a weekend away with friends) set up a host of problems.

In my second birth, even though I was prepared for this, I still found it hard to maintain the sacredness after our son was born. In fact, in both births, I found it much harder after the birth than during it.

If you are having problems (such as colic, mastitis, inability to cope with sleepless nights), it is a sign that you need to close the door and tune in with your baby, to reconnect and recreate the bubble.

It is so important to set up some support system (child care for other children, a cook delivering delicious meals etc) ready for this most precious time, and stay in the bubble for a good 40 days allowing you to be nurtures as you nurture your baby to gently incarnate.

It is always good to have some healing in the form of Reiki and cranial sacral therapy for both mother and baby to ease this transition, whilst clearing any twists that might have occurred in the birth itself.

If you have other children, this is sacred time to initiate bonding between them. The first meeting will impact their future relationships. Try to have the room quiet and all other people removed – including the father, possibly - so that, as mother, you can welcome your other child and then introduce him/her to the baby.

After the birth, close the space simply and quickly by asking for grounding and protection. Give thanks for what has happened and ask for continued protection in the early days to come, for the highest good of all concerned. Cover your head for a few days/weeks, to ground yourself.

Vitamin K

Vitamin K is given routinely to babies in the UK, although not in many other countries such as Canada. It is given to prevent internal bleeding, which can be a risk in very rare circumstances. The risk is slightly elevated if the baby has experienced a traumatic birth. Consider whether this is necessary for your child. It can be given via injection or oral drops, but both of these have been implicated in producing side effects which can be long-lasting and many people refuse it as unnecessary. Research your options and make your decisions clear.

Vaccination

The routine vaccination schedule in the UK begins at eight weeks of age and includes more than twelve injections before the age of thirteen months, many of which include vaccinations against multiple diseases. This is a medical intervention and vaccinations can cause serious life long side effects, including brain damage, cot death and autism. Many people feel that vaccines do not offer the protection they claim to, since many people contract illnesses they have been vaccinated against. It is very difficult these days to obtain objective information about the safety and effectiveness of vaccinations because anything that goes against the pharmaceutical profit making organisations is removed or labelled misinformation. It is very important to consider this subject carefully. The Arnica organisation (www.Arnica.org.uk) or The Informed Parent (www.informedparent.co.uk) can provide links to research that will help you to make a more informed decision. Even if you decide to vaccinate your child, the benefits of delaying the vaccinations are vital to consider.

Learning from other Cultures

In some cultures, babies do not leave their birthing space for forty days to give their soul time to incarnate. They are then gently and slowly taken into the community. Many people do not believe in having extended family, friends or visitors of any kind for the first few weeks.

"After giving birth both mothers and baby are thought to be at special risk, the mother because of her exertions and the subsequent weakening of her body, and the baby because of the sudden change in environment and possibility that his or her soul is not yet firmly established in the body." Jacqueline. Vincent Priya.

Most traditional cultures have common ways of taking care of the mother and baby which include:

Exclusion of normal duties for at least forty days

To be treated like queens during the rest and recovery stage, remaining at home for forty days or more to rest and get strong again, to enable breast (heart) feeding to be properly established

Daily massage and abdominal binding for the mother

Use of medicinal herbs

Mother heating on a special platform or by fires to keep her warm

Simple warming food

Few visitors are allowed

Baby and mother avoid extreme sensations at all costs: noise, weather etc.

"The majority of births occur in the warmer months of summer. For one whole week after his baby is born, the father avoids working in the fields for fear of inadvertently harming even the smallest insect, and thus disturbing the ihu. *Mother and child remain peacefully in a separate room, protected from the outside world. The family spoils them, bringing the freshest and richest milk, and the best yak butter. They hang an arrow of good fortune from the willow ribbed ceiling. So long as the* onpo *gives his approval, it is on the seventh day that neighbours and friends are invited to see the newborn child for the first time. They come with heaped plates of flour and butter, and little figures moulded from dough in the shape of an ibex, the Horse of the Gods.*

In the prayer room, monks burn incense. The house echoes to the hypnotic sounds of plainsong chant, and the harsh reedy tones of the religious music…

The celebrations that take place a month after the birth involve the whole village. A child has been born to the community. The blacksmith comes with gifts of a spoon and bracelet. The musicians play a lharnga. Kataks *and special food are brought for the mother and child.*

The onpo *also chooses the day on which the baby should leave the house for the first time. Nothing is left to chance. All the omens must be favourable and the elements especially well matched.*

The parents rub a little butter on the baby's head for good luck, and paint a black mark of soot and oil, jur, *on the forehead, to ward off evil spirits. They dress it in a long homespun robe and a woollen hat adorned with a silver* om.

After two or three months, the baby is taken to the monastery to be blessed and given a printed prayer for protection. It is at this time too that the infant receives what we would consider first names from a rinpoche *or high lama. The names are derived from Buddhist concepts; for example "angchuk" and "wangyal" " mean "powerful" and "victorious" in the sense of overcoming one's ego…"*

Ancient Futures, Learning From Ladakh
Helena Norberg-Hodge

Welcoming your Baby Exercise

Based on what you have just read, spend some time now thinking about questions such as:
What can you do to welcome your baby?
What does it feel like to be a newborn baby?
What steps can you take now to protect your baby's space after the birth?
The book "You are Your Child's First Teacher" by Rahima Bladwin Dancy has an excellent first chapter entitled "Receiving and Caring for the Newborn" which can help you with the preparation for these first few weeks. This is an excellent book to support you as a parent too.

A Ceremony for Welcoming and Blessing your Baby

No matter how you birthed or what the outcome, this is an important part of closing your birth and entering the world. It is an important part of stage four of the birth. I recommend doing the ceremony privately alone with baby and your children and partner at first. You can always do another more public one later. This is a sacred ceremony, to anchor and bless and welcome in your incarnating baby. It is for all of you too.

You may want to use the placenta/after birth as part of this ritual. It may be the first time you and your baby leave the house together with the sacred cloth that you wrapped around your baby after he/she was born. This may even be a naming ceremony for just you, your partner and your baby – or you may want to invite others along.

In a power place or special place for you all, take the placenta and your baby and some crystals, incense, candles, white feathers and things that have meant something to you during pregnancy and birth or been on your birthing altar.

After setting the space and grounding and protecting (white and golden light and red roots), invoke the sacred beings that helped you to birth.
Name the qualities that you thank them for.
Bless your baby and name the qualities that you invoke for your baby's life.
Name your baby if you are ready to do so.
Bury the placenta if you want to do so, or you may prefer to take it home and eat it or dry it and grind it into alchemical medicine.
Bless your baby and welcome your baby with spring water or a kiss.
Give thanks and close the ceremony.

For the highest good of all concerned, your baby is blessed and welcomed! So Be It and so it is!

Congratulations!

Post Natal Care for the Mother's Body

Mantra with visualisation and letting go to God. *My birth and woman tissues are returning to their normal way of being, easily, effortlessly, gently and healthily, I am a hundred times healthier than I was before!* Visualise and affirm during feed times that the uterus returns to normal and all the tissues knit together perfectly. *I am more healthy than ever before! This birth has healed my body and filled it with light!*

Fear release and tension release. Even if you think you do not need to do this, you have gone through a huge event which will be stored in your body. Keep focused on the mantras that you have been doing and have postnatal ones prepared beforehand for use while doing tension release, focusing on your shoulders and jaw.

Homeopathy for five days:
Do your own research or see a Practitioner. Common remedies include:
Arnica 200c twice daily.
Arnica 30c, Hypericum 30c, Bellis Perennis 30c, take all 3 at same time, 3x a day to reduce pain and swelling.
Calendula 30c, take one hour after birth for tears.
Chamomilla 30c, twice a day for after sensations whilst feeding.
Kali phos 30c, 1 dose for exhaustion and sleep.

Vitamins and Nutrition Floradix, hemp or linseed oil, superfoods, hot water and lemon, fennel tea, Siberian ginseng tonic, raspberry leaf/nettles/squawvine/crampbark tea. Continue avoiding wheat and sugar and eat vegetable soups etc.

Rescue remedy Use regularly and stroke baby's aura with it diluted in water.

Washing Use water with salt alongside Calendula/Hypericum tincture. Try mixing the salt with almond oil, essential oils (for example, Mother Amma has a lovely rose oil which she has blessed) and lavender/rose petals. Put chamomile teabags in the bath.

Reflexology and Massage or Reiki for mother and baby. Massage yourself daily with Rose Otto (and/or get someone to massage you). Massage your baby by stroking his/her aura with rescue remedy and washing the cord in chamomile tea. Many new mothers tend to be hunched over with tension and protection for their baby, as well as from all the lifting and feeding, not to mention the birth itself. In some cultures, new mothers are massaged **daily** and given hot sweats. Make a list of things that will support you: friends, parental counsellors, parenting books and organisations, websites, magazines, therapists, etc.

Cranial Sacral Therapy for baby and mother to realign the spine following birth and trauma.

Exercise Pelvic floor exercises, deep breathing, ankle and abdominal exercises.

Summary –
Tools For Maintaining A Clear Post Natal Period

1. Placenta – give it time.
2. Cutting cord – again, give it time. Do I want to cut it or leave it on for a few days to do its own thing?
3. Holding the space and not tidying it all away.

4. Quiet and candlelit.
5. Breast feeding.
6. Massage.
7. Intimate space – left alone, maintain privacy.
8. Having a sacred birth cloth or blanket ready to wrap my baby.
9. Having a cook to bring meals daily for us all

Add more of your own here....

Birth Acceptance and Birth Healing

You can use this section to accept your birth (whether you had the birth you wished for or not) for releasing any birthing issues or for healing traumatic outcomes.

Birth is no goal to achieve - you are not a success or a failure depending on how smooth or painful your birth was. The baby has its own karma and the birth will affect the persona and karma they need to create for their life's lessons. You can never judge your own (or another person's) birth.

If you feel your birth went "wrong", you need to ask yourself, "is this really wrong? Or is there a great lesson in this?" You may not be able to understand the lesson right now, it may be that you look back in twenty years and say "wow! That birth was so like her!"

What is "wrong" if everything that happens is in accord with the divine plan? If you follow your instincts, then you will have the birth that you and your baby are meant to have. Remember, your baby has its own karma and path to follow which is out of your hands. This is important to remember in any outcome that does not suit you. Your baby's soul has its own plan and reasons for coming the way that it comes. If you let go and surrender to your baby and your body and follow the energy, everything will be happening exactly as it is meant to be.

"The fate of the soul is determined in accordance with its prarabdha-karma. What is not meant to happen will not happen, however much you wish it. What is meant to happen will happen, no matter what you do to prevent it. This is certain. Therefore the best path is to remain silent."
Ramana Maharshi (Indian sage)

There is no right or wrong birth, no birth is a success or a failure, all births are what they are meant to be.

If you feel any negative emotions towards your birth, however traumatic or not it might have been (or however long ago), remember, there are no accidents. Accidents are events that we attract to us to reflect any emotional states that we might carry within. Your birth is your mirror and you tend to birth as you live.

A traumatic birth can be one of the greatest teachers on the spiritual path. Work through your birth and learn from it. Were there any issues that you did not resolve? Can you resolve them now? Sometimes the more you heal, the more you have to heal. Like the layers of an onion, as you peel one back, another can emerge. Things you never knew were lurking may crop up.

Loving yourself as a human means forgiving yourself and accepting. You can say "oh ok, I get it", and move onto the next lesson on the next rung of the ladder of your spiritual pathway.

Do the forgiveness exercise in this book. In this way you can thank any events that have been traumatic and any people that have presented challenges for you, as mirrors and teachers for the pathway to inner growth and peace. Forgive yourself as well for not having resolved any issues at the birth time.

We think birth should be like this ... but actually it is a reflection of you and your baby's "dharma". It is what is, or it was what was. Here-in lies acceptance in the practise of non judgement.

Things also happen for many unknown reasons, not just as part of your journey to learn what you need to learn. Remember that you cannot always perceive your best interests as you do not have all the information to hand. For example, some people say that a specific type of crystal child will be born with a big head and often may need a caesarean section.

A Course in Miracles says that we do not have all the information. Only God and the angels know what you need to have. Remember the Good Luck-Bad Luck story in the Introduction? Or the anecdote about the birds in Step Ten of Part One? If you are in tune, and you have complications, maybe they were necessary for the highest good of all for an unknown reason.

Also remember that your baby's karma is involved too. How you both birth reflects and affects their karmic path in this lifetime. These are choices that they have made previous to incarnation. You may be responsible as mother for their emotional welfare, but you are not entirely responsible. Children choose you for their own lessons. The book "*Journey Of Souls: Case Studies of Life Between Lives*" by Ph.D. Michael Newton is a fascinating study of where souls go in between lives and why they incarnate and draw the births, lives, major events and people towards them and how it is all predestined for karmic lessons for the greatest good beyond our rational reckoning.

"You may house their bodies but not their souls, for their souls dwell in the house of tomorrow which you cannot visit, not even in your dreams"
The Prophet, Kahil Kibran

The way a baby is born relates to their personalities. If birth is the first step on the parenting ladder and each step affects the other, we can see that a baby chooses their birth just as they choose their parents. Both are instrumental to their future life. If the birth affects your baby's personality then the birth is already written into the cosmos as part of your baby's horoscope? So you can let go and know that all is as it is meant to be and everything is part of the divine plan. Do not use this as an excuse to give up on manifestation for an imminent birth, though! Your manifestation plan is also part of the divine plan as your baby has chosen you to manifest the right birth for them. Just tune in well, as explained in part one.

There is a story about Shirdi Sai Baba that goes as follows:

A woman's son was bitten by a cobra and she begged Shirdi Sai Baba for sacred ash to heal it, but he refused and the son died. Seeing her immense grief, one of his devotees begged him
"Please Baba, for my sake, revive her son" but he replied,
"Don't get involved in this. What has happened is for the best. Her son's soul has already entered another body, in which he can do especially good work – work that he could not do in this one. If I draw him back into this body, the new one he has entered will have to die in order for this one to love. I might do it for your sake, but have you considered the consequences? Have you any idea of the responsibility, and are you prepared to assume it?"

The 4 Step Birth Fear Release Action Plan

1   Use personal unique mantra or affirmation after going quantum in ways outlined in Part One. Refer to the fear release action plan. If you had a traumatic birth you could ask "why did I attract that event?" " Even if it was not traumatic, you may still feel that you want to release some 'stuff'

2   Use Visualisation. Refer to the birth release meditation below.

3   Have cranial sacral treatments (and other therapies) to aid the transition and release trauma in the body alignment. It is never too late to do this for both of you, even if your baby is now ten years old.

4   Fuse acceptance and forgiveness. Follow the birth acceptance exercise below. Refer to the manifestation plan and follow the exercises on acceptance and forgiveness for yourself, your baby, your body and all those who were involved.

Birth Acceptance Exercise

Everything is perfect as it is. When you walk in the woods you do not wish that the oak were an elm.

"My birth should have been… my child should be … my partner should… if you loved me you would …. If I had … I would have…"

Take half an hour to really focus on everything being perfect as it is without judgement and spend the rest of the day consciously applying this idea to your birth.

"Give each incarnation the space to manifest exactly as it needs to manifest"
Ram Dass.

See the perfection in seemingly "wrong" situations, see the divine flow in everything.

Birth Release Meditation

Close your eyes and take some deep breaths in a relaxed place at a time when you can be assured of 20 minutes or more of uninterrupted time.

Ask for holding and grounding.

Return to your garden and sit upon your safe chair.

Deeply relax.

Ask your guides and angels to be present alongside your Higher Self and your baby's Guides, Angels and Higher Self, for the highest good of all concerned.

State that you request birth release and birth healing where appropriate to occur right now.

Ask your Angels and Guides to go back in time to release any pain and heal any trauma for all concerned in the birthing space. Right now.

Send Christ light back in time to your birth and to where you feel you needed it most. Send yourself healing and love and then send it to your baby. Really take time to do this. Now tune into the Divine Mother image on the back of this book and feel her love and her messages and that the divine plan is happening for the highest good of all.

Now go through the entire birth again in detail, in your mind's eye and tune into the parts of your birth which you feel were traumatic. There may be things that arise that you had not thought of as a problem at the time and vice versa – things that you thought were traumatic may not have been so.

Ask your Guides and your heart for answers to any questions you might have about this. When you have spoken to them, send further love and healing to your body and baby by shining light, thanking your body and baby for all that they did and ask for all trauma to be released right now. See it healing and releasing. As you shine Light onto the sticky parts of it, or any parts that make you feel unhappy or tense, know that time is not linear and that as you do this it is corrected.

Do the same now from your baby's point of view: go through the birth as if you were your baby and shine Light on all parts of it where your baby may feel tense.

Then ask for acceptance and forgive anyone you might need to. Send love to any other people who were present and say to them "I release and forgive you. I know that you were merely following your own journey in life and no longer hold any resentments towards you. I forgive you and I let you go as I forgive myself and let myself go from this situation."

There might be sensations or events that you need to accept and send love towards. You can now accept any traumatic events and also change them if needs be. For example, if you felt that the cord was cut too early, you can now return to this place and send loving energy and a feeling of time and space to it, imagining that the trauma is released and it no longer matters.

Talk to your baby now and see if they need anything – healing, therapy, words, colour etc. to heal them and help them release any birth trauma. Send them Christ light and colours that heal. Talk to your baby's higher self. See them in a rainbow garden, and ask them if they have any messages for you.

Once you feel that you have healed and breathed light into your birth and released all the trauma into the light for healing, you can give thanks and return from your garden.

Affirm "My birth is now healed. Even though this ... happened, it is ok and I now accept this and feel no trauma about it since it has been released to the light. I see this event as a positive one and surround it with loving light. Now, when I think of this event, it heals and strengthens me! I feel happy about it and draw peace from it. From now onwards, I will always see this event as a positive healing experience. I am now at peace with the events that occurred during my birth and I let all resentments dissipate into the light. I forgive and I accept right now. My baby and I are healed. I really see this and know this right now. From now onwards, I think of my birth with only love and happiness, knowing all is well and healed and all occurred that needed to for the highest good of all concerned."

Visualise your birth surrounded by light right now.

Breathe in the light that now surrounds your birth, sending healing vibrations to the past and the present for both you and your baby. Know that time is not linear and that you can affect and heal the past by sending love to it from the future.

Give thanks.

Examples of Postnatal Mantras

When sleep deprived with a breast fed baby, it is easy to descend into mental fog. Breastfed babies get hungry more quickly than formula fed babies since formula slows down the digestive process so breastfeeding can feel constant to begin with. The early days are testing times.

These affirmations can remind you that you choose to sink or rise, for clarity or fog.

Keep up with your other affirmations and do them as much as you can. Really feel and imagine what you are saying: remember, intent and emotion are everything, use words which come from you subconscious and not your mind.

My children are divinely protected and surrounded by love.
I rise and remain on top of things.
I know.
I am fully in power and easily attend to my baby's needs whilst easily attending to my needs too.
I have enough time for my relationship.
I have the energy to listen to my needs as well as those of my baby and relationship. Easily.
I am fully whole and in power.
I am able. I am able to walk tall. I am able to be free.
I am fully supported and the universe provides me with all that I need at the right time. All I need to do is ASK then ACT "AS IF", KNOWING.
I CHOOSE self power.
I CHOOSE energy and space.
I CHOOSE to guide my own life from within me, from source.
I CHOOSE to be energised.
I CHOOSE a positive mindset towards my children and towards being a parent of children with need to be met.
I welcome my children's needs since I welcome my children (they are after all well come).

I look within to God for my needs to be met – God is my source.
All is well in the eyes of God.
I have time and space for all the things that I want.
I relax.
I surrender.
I have a chilled out attitude towards parenting.
My baby thrives, my baby is well.
At any time when my baby needs me I will be there as my inner knowing is deeply in tune with my baby and I trust it.
I let go and have faith in God that all is well for my baby.
I am able to easily nourish and attend to my baby's needs throughout the night as required. When my baby awakes I feel happy to nourish him and fall back into restful sleep again afterwards.
I feel youthful and young and vibrant.
My children empower me and give me new life, we have fun!
I love being a mother, it suits me well.
I relax into motherhood.
I take each day as it comes and somehow or another manage to get enough rest so that I am able to meet the needs of myself and my children.
My children flow and dance well together in all that they do.
My children are deeply loved.
Even though I carry a baby/have lots of children, my hands are still free and I am able and fit.
God provides all I need.
I can do it easily and effortlessly.
All is well.
I am the source.

Play around with changing the tenses from past to present and from "I" to "you" as you read each one out. Remember to **allow** and **flow**, rather than "mind impose". These are examples, find the ones that come from or resonate with your own subconscious.

7 - Clear Parent

Intuitive Parenting Techniques for Stage Four and Beyond

"The most powerful prayer is the prayer of the Mother"
Yogi Bhajan

"Women have millions of years of genetically-encoded intelligences, intuitions, capacities, knowledges, powers, and cellular knowledge of exactly what to do with the infant."
Joseph Chilton Pearce

'Intuitive Parenting' is a big part of 'Intuitive Birthing'. If you already have a child, you need to be able to create a space of practising self love whilst simultaneously parenting and meeting everyone's needs, in order to prepare for a relaxed birth. If you are in a tense parent space, how can you birth in a relaxed way? If you do not have children yet, thinking about how you will meet your own needs, those of your relationship and those of your baby is an important task for now, not for later.

When I had our first baby, I was in shock afterwards as I had spent so long preparing for the birth that I had forgotten about preparing for a baby! Having a home birth meant that as soon as the birth was over, I was left alone with my baby and no help. I was forced into a place of trusting myself and my own instincts, having few friends around with babies as I was the first of my friends to have one. I found myself parenting in ways I never would have expected as my baby seemed to have her own agenda and the birth also continued into the parenting space with its sacred flow.

Following Sacred birthing, the next natural progression is sacred parenting with intuitive techniques. What would that mean for you and do you have the support around to follow these instincts? For example, when you have a sacred birth and go immediately into responsive breastfeeding (feeding on demand), you will naturally find that your baby will not be put down easily and it will feel wrong to put your baby in another room.

You may prefer to have your baby in your bed so that she/he undergoes an easier incarnation transition from womb to outer form and as it is so much easier to remain nourished during night time feeds if you do not have to keep getting up. What a wonderful gift for a newborn baby to sleep with its mother, feeding in a snug, womblike environment and reconnecting whenever it needs to. Pregnant women are hit with marketing for baby gadgets which actually are mostly unnecessary, you can have your baby in your bed and carry her in your arms and change her on a soft rug - these prams and cots and tables are not necessary! It is often a relief to remove yourself from all that marketing and come into a place of stillness and nature.

However, if you want your baby to have its own space as well, a solution may be a bedside cot, you can get round ones that are womb like with no sharp edges, on wheels (good for rocking) and with a detachable side. Bedside cots go right next to you and you can roll to feed your baby on your side or slide your baby into the cot whilst they also get used to their own space. Cleanse the area and fill it with beautiful, handmade, natural things like lavender bags that you and your children have made by hand and filled with light. Bless the space and place a Guardian Angel there.

Like this example of co–sleeping, there are many ways of finding a balance in meeting everyone's needs. Beware of following parenting methods as they simply cannot be applied to everyone since we are all unique. Like Intuitive Birthing, Intuitive Parenting is about **deepening our connection** with both ourselves and our children so that we can more easily access and meet everyone's needs. Intuitive Parenting is based on the understanding that **we are all unique and all our situations are unique.**

In Intuitive Birthing, nothing is wrong. Home births are advocated as it is easier to follow your instincts and set up a sacred space at home than in a hospital. Similarly, although there is no "right" or "more sacred" way to parent, it is easier to hear and apply intuitive techniques with 'attachment' parenting principles - co-sleeping, prolonged breastfeeding, sling wearing, conscious communication, positive discipline. Intuitive Parenting means exploring ways and means that are gradual and gentle, rather than methods that are traumatic, to achieve the same result (i.e. to get your baby sleeping). At the same time though, Intuitive Parenting does not advocate these attachment parenting connection techniques as the only way. You need to use your intuition to find the best solution for your baby and yourself.

When you are a new parent, you have to balance many needs and approaches and apply them in a trial and error way… Let's apply Intuitive Parenting to sleeping, as an example. As opposed to traumatic sleep training methods, Intuitive Parenting promotes using "rhythm" as opposed to "schedule": allowing your baby to sleep, rather than imposing on him to sleep. Do you have to clock watch? Could you follow a flow rather than an order? How often, when you *'let it go'* and don't mind, does your baby fall asleep anyway?! Remember the fundamental truths in this book for manifestation in such times: acting "as if".

So watch your attitude towards allowing: does it matter if your baby does not sleep through if you can catch up at other times? You only have a baby for a short moment in a lifetime. It can be about understanding facts: did you know that a breastfed baby digests milk quicker and needs to wake more often? It can be about trust: trust that your baby knows what he is doing, whilst nudging him or her gently to be in the direction that is best for your family. It is about juggling things around and getting help so that you can sleep. But beyond all of these things, **it is about employing the manifestation and affirmation techniques in this book to create the situation you want, whilst being in tune with your family (using the visualisations), so that you can allow the highest good to occur for all**. Intuitive Parenting employs all the things you have learnt about presence, intuition and higher self and applies them to parenting.

Keep on looking at and doing the Divine Mother Meditation so you can remain in the flow of this harmonious vibration.

The basis of intuitive parenting rests in **self nourishment** so that you can hear your intuition. It draws upon part of Rudolf Steiner's philosophy, which teaches that children learn through imitation so our *words* and *actions* are very important. Intuitive parenting means that you can be child aware and avoid traumatic techniques such as "crying it out" whilst remembering yourself. Many mothers drawn to sacred parenting become "child-led", yet for a child to be happy in a healthy home and healthy marriage, all must be rooted in your relationship with yourself and remembering yourself.

We can look to traditional societies for guidance in Intuitive Parenting as well as Intuitive birth:

"They have continual physical contact with others, a factor that plays an important role in their development. Dolma spent more time with little angchuk, who was six months old, than anyone else did. All night he would sleep in her arms, able to feed whenever he wanted. In the daytime she would usually take him with her if she was working in the fields. But caring for her baby was not her job alone. Everyone looked after him…
The traditional way of life allows mother and children to remain together at all times. When villagers gather to discuss important issues, or at festivals and parties, children are always present. Even at social gatherings that run late into the night with drinking, singing, dancing and loud music, young children are seen running around, joining the festivities until they simply drop off to sleep. No one tells them "It's eight thirty. You must be off to bed".
I told Dolma how much time babies in the West spend away from their mothers and how at night they might sleep in another room and be fed cow's milk from plastic bottles on a schedule rather than when they cry. She was horrified: "Please, atche Helena, when you have children, whatever you do, don't treat your baby like that. If you want a happy baby, do like we do."
Ancient Futures, Learning From Ladakh By Helena Norberg-Hodge.

Co-sleeping, prolonged breast-feeding, tandem-feeding are all methods that really hold children and allow them to be nourished deeply at a soul level. Childhood is not a race to the finishing line. Sacred parented children may not be ready to flee the nest as early as other children but when they are truly ready to, they will do so from a held and rooted security and have less problems in adolescence.

At the same time, we do not live in a culture that has the community resources to support this method of parenting much yet. Following attachment parenting with co sleeping, prolonged breastfeeding and tandem nursing can really support you and make things easier, but it can also easily lead to exhaustion from having a lack of support: from mind imposing rather than tuning in. Doing it differently can be threatening to others, and then in turn create a rigid approach that acts in defiance of traditional approaches, causing alienation from community and family and even friends. An 'us' and 'them' situation arises. It is at such times that we really need to put the methods in this book into practise.

"It's hard sometimes being raw in a cooked world, being holistic in a medical world, being conscious in a pretty unconscious world, being attached in a disconnected detached world".
Laura M in email to the "raw mom summit"

"The expectations and the standards put out there by these speakers are ridiculous! I am a health-conscious mom of two beautiful kids who I've nursed, co-slept with, haven't vaccinated, treated with homeopathy, etc. I "get it". I've been curious about the "raw food diet" and the "raw food lifestyle" but after listening to these calls, I do not feel encouraged to adopt this lifestyle! Instead, I want to tell everyone to lighten up! I want my kids to be truly healthy. As in, I want them to be able to cope well with any situation they are presented with. I really don't see how severely restricting their diet, isolating them from other kids their age, and taking them out of places where they want to be like their friends is setting them up to be well-rounded kids. Of course, I want to protect them from the dangers of the world, including foods that may poison them. But I don't want them to be afraid of the world. They will survive a glass of milk here and there. They will survive a

sandwich. They will even survive a piece of pizza. And in the end, they might be better for it, actually. Thanks, K."
Anonymous woman's email to the raw food summit.

After my second birth, after some research, I decided to tandem feed as my first baby was not yet ready to wean. Breastfeeding throughout the pregnancy and second birth itself was a joyful experience, but as soon as my baby arrived, I couldn't bear to breastfeed my toddler. The strong negative emotions overwhelmed me and my toddler. I created the very experience of sibling rivalry that I was trying to avoid, the reason I had decided to tandem feed in the first place! I wrote to some sacred parenting organisations for support but felt more pressure from these places to continue to tandem feed. In the end, I became ill with scarlet fever, which led to an extreme prolonged skin rash, hospital treatment and chronic fatigue and my family (parents) had to pick up the pieces. They parent in more old-fashioned ways with television, sleep training and so on. But during this time I learnt to accept the importance of balance. I had to relax and be open to everything, without judgement. It was a powerful lesson indeed.

Sol learnt more about what Intuitive Parenting is really about: being a clear channel so that you can do what is right for you, rather than following someone else's ideas or imposing your own ideals. I realised that I had actually been 'anxiety parenting' when I thought I was 'holistically parenting' and my meditations from the wonderful birth went out of the window when I was busy with babies. I forgot how to 'let go'.

In summary therefore, Intuitive Parenting means employing the techniques in this book and applying them to parenting: remembering and developing mantras, doing meditations, having healing, massages and so on, basically looking after yourself well and staying tuned in and relaxed. So here are a few exercises for Intuitive Parenting that I hope you may find helpful:

Exercise for Parenting Approach

Ask yourself:
What can I give my children? What is my intuitive feeling on where to put my baby to sleep? How can I talk to my child if she does something inappropriate? What are my feelings on long term breastfeeding?

Whilst you cannot possibly know and account for future situations, it is also a positive thing to start considering your approaches now. Check into your intuition using the visualisations in this book.

You need to start thinking about tuning into the highest good for yourself, starting sentences with "I love myself therefore…", alongside tuning into the highest good for all members of your immediate family, starting sentences with "I love my baby/husband therefore…." as well.

Write questions and answers in your journal, such as the example below.

Q. What do my children need that traditional parenting does not offer?

A. Heart, presence, awareness of consequences, positive language, connection - as opposed to coercion and threats and power struggles over food (try smoothies and healthy nibbles).

Relationships are the foundation for emotions my children will respond and mirror when forming their personality... to heal and release trauma and resentments and hurts I carry ...

Visualisation for Healthy Breastfeeding

When you first try and breastfeed it can be a bit odd, and lots of 'head' thoughts come into interfere with the "latch on" which is new to you both. Phrases like "nose to nipple" and "has she got enough of the nipple in there?" can confuse the process. Then one is encouraged to think about positioning techniques and ends up in conversations about setting a breastfeeding space and time, or doing it just on demand, whilst worrying, "am I giving equally from both breasts? Should I give more foremilk first on my left breast?" and so on....Wow! It is no wonder breast feeding issues exist - all this after a birth and with very little sleep!

The best way to breastfeed well is to forget about all of that, and instead just know that it is fine. New babies take their time, hours, days, weeks, to adjust and may not know how to suckle immediately and that's just fine.

Close your eyes now.
Take some breaths.
Don't control your breathing, just watch it.
Relax.
Forget all about right and wrong. Just relax.
Now imagine your baby healthy and strong, feeding from you well. Imagine feeding your baby in abundance and you producing the right amount of milk easily whilst feeling energised! Imagine your language, what you say to people in passing about how easy you have found it and so on. Feel what this feels like.
Now let your body know that this is how it is for you and your baby. Tell your body that this is the situation and that nothing else will be listened to, this is your story now. Choose this story now as yours.
Really be clear with the feeding.
Tell your body that it knows what to do, like birthing or menstrual bleeding, your body will just keep on being a woman and will provide beautiful milk for your baby.

You let go and trust your baby and your body.

Your milk flows from your heart. As you feed your baby, you feed from your heart and your baby fills up on energy from their vortex of creation. You are their channel to God and your milk is God light for your baby. What you think and feel, your baby will think and feel too. Ensure that as you feed you do so in calm, quiet, loving ways with positive visual imaginings in your head and using positive language. Use colour and see yourselves surrounded by protective and healing lights. Use mantras and yogic exercises to heal your heart to purify your breast milk.

Repeat I LOVE I LOVE I LOVE I AM SURROUNDED BY LOVE. Really feel this.

Now do not bother with conversations or thoughts of times and latches and foremilks. Yes, you may want to check which breast is bigger, but let go to your body, to your baby and most of all to your intuition.

Your breast milk is beautiful and your baby is getting strong and healthy. You are amazing at breastfeeding. You feed with abundance. This is your story from now onwards.

So be it and so it is for the highest good of all concerned, Amen.

Meditation for Being Present with your Child

You can do this anytime: when breastfeeding or weaning, when playing or before going to sleep. You could do this if your child is absent, just imagine them with you if you want to connect to them, or if your child is hurting. If the latter is the case, they will probably calm down as you do it but do not hold onto the goal of calming them down.

Sit with your child on your lap.
Take some deep breaths, they may copy you.
Breathe in light and as you breathe out let tension drain out of your feet.
Ask for love to be present.
Imagine a bubble of love surrounding you both, protecting you.
You can then imagine a figure of eight encircling you both. Whilst your baby is protected in pink light, the figure of eight protects you in blue. Keep the figure of eight going so that you are joined and protected but in your own spaces.
Breathe in light and, as you breathe out, breathe light out, shining it and radiating it from you into your child and all around you.
Breathe in light and breathe it from your heart into theirs.
Imagine light connecting you from your heart to theirs.
This light can stretch across continents.
You may want to look into their eyes or let them rest their head against your chest as you kiss the top of their head.
Really feel the connection and just be in it in silence, talking quietly, reading a book or saying a mantra of love or "Om". Keep returning to the heart connection in your mind's eye. You may want to see this as a colour, either green or pink.
You can ask for your child's protection from a goddess of your choice.
They will run off when they have finished or you will draw it to an end naturally. You can do this for as little as half a minute or as much as twenty minutes or more.
Afterwards keep imagining the love that engulfs you and your child whenever you feel like it and know that they are safe and feel loved deep inside.

Note: You may sense a voice inside that is your baby's Higher Self communicating its needs. You will know if this is projection or if it is your baby's Higher Self. Be confident in this if it happens and do not dismiss it as just your imagination as your baby can communicate a lot to you in this way.

Calming an Anxious Baby

If your baby is anxious or ill, you need to tune in to yourself first to see where you are at. Focus on being centred as much as you can so that you can be in tune with your intuition. This is essential for your baby, and your baby will draw nourishment from your place of power and connection and from your own nourishment.

Tune in and see what you are fearful of and if there are any blocks then use affirmations by following the ten steps in part one. Say them to your baby regularly like a mantra and really imagine them as you say them. *"My baby is divinely protected and surrounded by love"*. Use the fear release action plan.

Keep on working on yourself, as you and your baby are one.

Breathe deeply. Shake out tension. Roll your shoulders. Relax, relax, relax. Use the Clear Channel of Light Meditation and keep breathing the light into you with a mantra to help you be calm. Watch how your baby's anxiety eases.

Use visualisation and talk to your baby's higher self to see if they have any messages for you.

Follow your inner knowingness, whatever arises and however strange it may feel, just go with it. For example, you may need to imagine the cord between you and your baby still being there and glowing with light. Whilst you do this and breathe with the visualisation, you may find your baby releases her/his anxiety.

Look at your Divine Mother image and feel the peaceful and safe vibration to calm things for you both.

Tune into your Higher Beings and Guides for guidance. Give offerings to God alongside angelic healing. Above all, keep thinking and imagining positive thoughts. You can do body healing on behalf of your baby too.

Meditation to Calm Mother and Child

You can ensure that you are acting from a clear place by connecting with this intuitive meditation.

If your child is insisting or having a tantrum, put down roots and ask for protection. Put roots down for your child and put protection lights around them too. Then ask for light for your child and light for yourself.

Keep breathing.

See the light come through your head and align you. Stay in this space with breaths. Keep breathing the light into your space and do not get caught in your child's pain.

When you feel strong and centred and able to remain in your truth you can then approach your child and help them align with the Light.

Connect with the Divine Mother image and feel the Divine Mother soft but very strong within at peace.

It is important that you are strong in your own space first when you approach your child, and stay in it when with your child. Then you can clearly decipher and tune into your intuition and act instinctually and clearly for the highest good of all. From this place of light you can listen to your child and not only get a sense of what is happening but also channel loving words that are needed for them at that time from a place of intuitive truth.

You may want to talk to them with loving mantras, put a healing hand onto their tummy or heart. Don't ask them to repress their feelings and do not be afraid of them letting out tension that needs to come out. It may be tension from something other than the current situation. Let them run their course whilst knowing that they are loved and supported enough to be able to express what they need to.

If they want something you cannot give, you might like to mirror their frustration with conscious communication, such as: *"this must feel…for you"*. State what it is, let them feel understood and heard.

Don't belittle it or tell them that it isn't, because it is for them. You might like to say *"I wish I could…but I can't and I know that this must feel…for you" "* using "I wish" is useful.

You may like to ask for or affirm peace on behalf of your child. You can affirm and manifest on behalf of another if you ask that it be in the highest good of all concerned and state that it is for them that you ask.

I am loved and I am light.
My child is divinely protected and surrounded by light.

Say this as a mantra.

All is well.
I am guided by God.
So be it and so it is.
For the highest good of all concerned.
Amen.

"The more you are able to follow your energy and do what is best for you, the more the universe will come through you to everyone around you. As you thrive, your children will too…We often have children that are spiritually more developed than we are so that we can learn from them…Our children essentially need two things from us:
1. They need to be recognised for who they really are. If we see that they are powerful and sophisticated spiritual beings and relate to them that way from the beginning, they will not need to hide their power and lose touch with their spirit, as most of us have. Their being will receive the support and acknowledgement they need to remain clear and strong.
*2. They need us to create an example for them of how to live effectively in the world of form. As we do this they watch how we live and imitate us. Being very perceptive and dogmatic, they copy what we actually **do** and not what we **say**."*

Shakti Gawain *Living in the Light.*

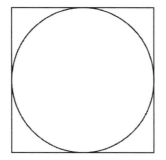

Part Three

Sacred Birth Manifestation

From Approximately Week 32

The Ten Step Birth Manifestation Action Plan

1.   Recreate your Birth Power Mantra Sheet in Part One. State clearly what you want.

2.   Relax and deep breathe, entering an altered state of consciousness, following the manifestation meditation.

3.   Release any blocks and then be in the Light. See yourself as happy whilst bathing in white Light.

4.   Ask the universe, then affirm daily, knowing that you are worthy of your desire. Speak the words, vocalising success using mantra/japa regularly through the day with "I am ..." sentences.

5.   Use visualisation. Imagine you have already achieved your goal; focus on how this feels, lingering on good feelings and using only positive thoughts and words. Have a drawing of your goal on the wall.

6.   Create opportunities whilst at the same time letting go and not worrying about HOW.

7.   Know and trust – act AS IF. Avoid people/places that drain you, or use protection. FEEL it as real in your body.

8.   Follow the energy and be aware of your thoughts.

9.   Be present. Be here now: as thought-aware and as thought-less as possible, seeing oneness in all other sentient beings and the abundance in the world. Start to drop the mantras and replace with seed mantras or silence, instead dwelling in just the positive feeling of the mantra, allowing the flow.

10.   Give thanks. For highest good of all concerned, so be it so it is. Then let it go. Once you have released it to the universe, you can trust that if things do not go your way then there is a reason and the universe has designs for you that are even greater than the ones that you conceived.

Forty Days to Manifest

Why forty days? According to most ancient traditions, religions and spiritual laws from all around the world, it takes forty days for your body to accept a new habit and take on a new way. However, if you read this book with less than forty days until your birth, please do continue.

We have talked about the need to be in a very clear place and a place of full power to enable birth and manifestation to take place. To be in the fullness of power means to be in a place of loving clear Light. Standing tall. Choosing abundance. If you live that truth then everything will work for you and your manifestation will occur. So keep on clearing out debris from yourself and your home, and keep on LOVING YOURSELF. It all starts with self love. Loving yourself means choosing self esteem and nourishment.

Now you have read this book and are in a clear place, you are ready to manifest!

Return to Part One and redo the ten steps to create your sacred birth power mantras alongside the Birth Rehearsal in the chapter on Clear Birth. The first time that you did this was a dress rehearsal. Now you know what to do and how it works, you can recreate your birthing mantras clearly. These will constantly change as new issues crop up and you may need to keep returning to Part One to re-address them, as well as continually referring to the Ten Step Emotional Clearance Chart.

Once you have your birthing mantra sheet laid out clearly, you can begin following the ten step Manifestation Action Plan. The first time you do this, do it as a ritual by following the Birth Manifestation Ceremony alongside the Manifestation Meditation below.

The forty day programme is as simple as this: after you have done the ritual, you need to spend time every day for forty days being present with your unique Sacred Birth Power Mantras that you discovered through the subconscious quantum fields in Part One of this book. Use Part 2 to get Clear. Use the manifestation chart as your guide.

Once your ritual is done, it is complete and it is out in the ethos being created. The work is done. The forty days are a reminder to yourself and the cosmos to further seal it - the main work is already done.

There are a few simple factors to enhance your programme:

1. Focus on the Mantras
As part of your daily reflection, you absolutely focus on the mantras whilst visualising them. You could read them, be with them or write them out repeatedly - whatever works for you. Or use the Daily Birth Preparation Exercise below as a basis. You might like to turn the mantras into a visualisation story. There is an example of a manifestation meditation at the end of this programme to help you with this. You may find you need to focus on just one particular mantra in this time, but do read all the others out. You can read out your dream birth on the inside sheet as well, as part of this practise, if you want to but this is not always necessary as the mantras are the essential part of the focus. Refer to The Law of

Decree in the Birth Manifestation Ceremony. Remember the emotion behind the mantra is what is important. Remember to use present tense too.

2. Find your Birthing Mantra

Find just one key mantra that really works for you or a key word that signals for you to open up and calm down on cue. It might be the name of a God, a happy memory, someone you love, a colour, or sentences that are simple and clear: *"I love, Ram, all is well, blue, Angels, my beautiful baby, I surrender easily and well, my body knows what to do …etc." "* Say this word constantly from now on to relax yourself and get used to it in preparation for using this word/phrase in birth with your spiral. Repeat it throughout the day (Japa).

3. Hold your Internal Space in Silence

Apart from working with your birth partner, do not tell everyone about your mantras and what you are doing as it will dissipate the energy. You can tell them about the programme you are following, but keep your mantras to yourself.

4. Become the Mantra

Aside from your daily focusing time, you will be continuously working with these mantras by having them around you so that you become/live/know them. If you feel like it, you can enhance this by hanging them up on a wall or on a birth altar with your birth drawings and other images that inspire you. Or you may like to refer to them on waking, or before sleeping, or carry them everywhere with you. You may like to record them onto an mp3 player and listen to them regularly or have your partner read them to you as part of your birth rehearsal. Then when you know them, you become them, the words fall away and the emotion and intent become reality for you now. No words. A meditation.

5. Keep Following other Birthing Exercises

During the daily reflection time, continue enjoying birthing exercises as a part of your morning pregnancy ritual. This morning ritual is an essential part of the forty day programme so keep it up. These exercises might be the ones contained within this book, or other physical or relaxation programs that you have encountered, or simply massaging your tummy. It does not matter what you do, just ensure that you take an hour a day to focus and enjoy giving to yourself and being with your birthing being and baby. Keep tuning in and following your instincts. Make the ritual personal to you. Refer to the exercise list in the contents.

A formula for your daily ritual is suggested at the beginning of this book in "How to read this book". An example routine for your day is also suggested below. The power of routine is that it sets greater energy to the work that you are doing: the regularity of the routine will allow the intention to impress itself onto the subconscious and the universe.

6. Keep Up

"Keep up and you will be kept up" Yogi Bhajan

Forty is a magical number. In some cultures, mothers and babies do not leave the house for forty days after birthing. It takes forty days for a truth to be realised energetically. Therefore, keep doing it every day. You can do this by having a 'start day' timetabled in your calendar. Whilst it is essential that you do not miss a day, it is also essential that you do not stress with "should". There may be some days where doing other exercises just seem too much and you need a break from them, in which case just do a massage. But don't get lazy: keep focused, keep using your intuition!

7. Readdressing New issues and Editing Your Birth Plan

If something arises and you need to re-address a feeling, simply return to Part One and use the exercises to resolve it, then add the new mantra to the forty day programme. There is usually no need for a new ritual. Keep it simple. Just say your intentions clearly and simply, then let them go. Do not get caught up in complicated and elaborate ongoing rituals with each new mantra. If you find yourself doing this then you need to return to trusting in the cosmos and yourself. Start to focus on believing your mantras so you can let them go, knowing "*All is well in the eyes of God*".

"All evil vanishes from life for him who keeps the sun in his heart"
(an old Hindu saying)

Birth Mantras from 32 Weeks

You have your own Mantras form you subconscious. These mantras are a guide for further inspiration to add from 32 weeks only. You may like to use any that resonate alongside your own - run you finger along them and feel them in you body to find the ones that leap out and shine for you, and discard any that do not.

I relax into sunshine and light daily
I empower myself in white light daily
My cervix is thinning daily
My baby glides out like a dolphin, healthy, strong, happy in a golden/white/pink/blue bubble of angel light
My baby is healthy, strong and protected
My body opens easily and comfortably
I can say yes to opening up wide as I am and I feel divinely protected, safe and surrounded by love
Fun, orgasmic, energising, beautiful ripples
I birth from mother river, safe and held
I birth from white light
My pelvic tissues and muscles are soft like jelly
I am safe in light
My body returns to a normal shape easily with hardly any bleeding
Birth is a healing gift for me, it is a secret of beauty!

"......For the highest good of all concerned, so be it and so it is, and now I let go".

Visualisation of Mantras

Make sure you address all issues you have, using positive language only (see Part One).

My baby is born from the Light dimension with Angels, Gods, Goddesses, Masters of Light and Ancient Midwives guiding us all.
We easily birth at home, magically and well, comfortably and happy, at ease for all of us... (name all members of family).
As we birth, the Angels watch and guide my other children as well so that their presence only contributes to the magic and ease of the birth. Our children are deeply connected and love and support each other in synchronicity and in rhythms of love with one another.
Our new baby glides out like a dolphin in the Light, dancing well with my body, and I surrender to my baby and my body and the cosmos. Safe to open wide. Safe to say Yes.

Opening easily and comfortably with beautiful ripples, easier than before. I choose now that it feels like this. I birth from the river mother in a space of Light.

The waves are watched by ... (name Angelic Beings and Spirit Guides). I feel beautiful and in my power as a woman like Aphrodite, I am protected by Artemis, and Mother Mary nourishes and lovingly guides and watches me and my children. My baby is guided by Master Angels such as…

My body knows how to birth and does it very well. My perineum is healthy, protected and safe at this time and heals easily.

After the birth, we have time and space to privately and safely and to gently and smoothly get to know each other and heal and ride our rhythms. My baby glides out of the Light healthy, strong and protected.

We are empowered in White Light every day.

A joyous celebration for us all.

For the highest good of all concerned, so be it and so it is.

Amen.

A Manifestation Meditation

In Section One we dived into manifestation and the power of thoughts as mantra when they comes from the subconscious or quantum field. The following meditation takes it one step further and can be used during or alongside the Birth Manifestation Ceremony. You may like to do it alone or with your partner. It is a meditation that focuses on the Law of Decree.

Close your eyes and relax with deep breaths.

Notice your breath, but do not change your breathing.

Just be with it.

Ask for grounding and holding.

Repeat your mantras as prayers, knowing that they are words of power. Choose a few that really work for you and keep on repeating them in a chant. Work alongside your breath.

Ask for any guides or beings of Light to be present and name them if you want, as well as your Higher Self and that of your baby.

Visualise your goals as if they are now. Really become the feeling as if it is true for you now.

Become it and do not entertain anything else from now on.

Sink deeply into the visualisation.

Now state your decree three times:

I decree in the name of love and light that….for the highest good of all concerned, so be it and so it is.

Amen.

Send love and light to yourself, your baby, and to the world.

Return, give thanks, let go and know that, from now on, it is so.

The Law of Decree unleashes great power, so make sure you are clear and sure in your words.

You might want to end your manifestation meditation with the words written by Julian of Norwich after an ecstatic vision on 13th May 1373:

All is well

And all will be well

And all manner of things will be well.

Examples of Pregnancy Daily Practises -

Christa's Pregnancy Daily Practise

Your pregnancy routine is approximately one hour a day. It is up to you if you want it to be any longer or shorter, somedays just 5 minutes is enough, other days you may want to deep dive. It is your positive choice to do this for yourself and your baby. Follow your intuition each day for exercises and time. If you want to do more than an hour a day, your daily timetable may look something like this:

Sat. 12th December

On waking in bed

- Practise instant relaxation with mantras and words that make me relaxed
- Listen to visualisation in bed or Light a candle and fill up with white Light and say my mantras. Imagine my placenta soft like jelly and talk to my baby to ask for easy birth whilst affirming position, and asking my cervix to open and thin out

This afternoon

- Yoga and body surrender

This evening

- Re-rehearse Birth rehearsal with John whilst doing the Perineum massage this evening. Would love some light touch massage (remind him I love it when he chants OM whilst putting his hands on my back!) Feeling worried about his workload; need to talk this through again, as well as doing a fear release and looking at affirmations to do with this issue. Also – relaxation script together every Sunday, or Saturday better??
- Relaxation meditation using colour before bed with key mantras.

Notes to self

NB. Read out mantras in my own voice to listen next week.

Also – Every time I go to the bathroom, remember to practise breath release with visualisation, as opposed to pushing! Likewise, practise mantras in queues in shops.

Example -
Christa's Birth Preparation Exercise

Monday's practise -
Open the circle, invoke Beings and ground, light candle.
Exercise - a shortened version of the Healthy Pregnant Body visualisation in Part Two.
Fill up with light by closing my eyes and taking deep breaths, imagining the healing white Light entering my head and washing me throughout. Tune in for messages. See a colour coming to cleanse me. Open my arms to the sunshine and let it into my heart. Breathe it in. Ask for Light then command it and affirm "I AM light".
Talk to my baby. Massage my belly. Send my baby and my body loving energy.
Recite my mantras.
Do some yoga from the other book, page 30, for half hour whilst listening to the Kundalini Yoga mantras on my phone.
Finally, ask for divine light circle three times and give a prayer of thanks.
Close the circle.

Once the 40 Days is up

Let go, surrender, allow!

Congratulations! Well done! Your birth is very near now and you can let go easily knowing that your "work" has been done. You can be confident and look forward to a beautiful and magical dream birth knowing that all is well and that you are guided.

If you want to, you can keep up with the "me" time, or you may feel like you need some time off to forget all about birth and babies and mantras now and just let go for a while and put it all aside to simply 'do its thing'.

Please remember to keep on following the flow and the energy. This means listening to your OWN instincts – do what you want and need to do. This might mean that you need to step away from your dream birth plan and do something unexpectedly different to that which you have imagined, do not impose your mind onto the flow. Even if the form differs slightly, the essence of your dream will manifest itself exactly as you have asked. If you let it go and follow your instincts, the form may be better than you could ever have dreamt it.

Keep remembering the Good Luck- Bad Luck story in the introduction: we do not have all the information so we cannot perceive our best interests. A seemingly bad situation could be ironically instrumental in making our dream birth occur or/and necessary for our baby's future life for some unknown reason.

'Success' (whatever that is for you) depends on following the Light. In an interview, Phillippe Pettit, the man who walked a tight rope between the twin towers in New York, says that in the lead up to the event he never once thought about the negatives: dying, being arrested and locked up... This was all irrelevant. The only thing of relevance was the magic of it working well and this was the ONLY thing he focused upon.

Finally, remember that the irony is that none of this stuff matters! All you need to do is be present in the here and now by letting it all go, right now, and relaxing. As discussed in the introduction: give up the craving for a desire and the desire will manifest anyway.

7 Key Pointers for Manifesting your Sacred Birth

1. Be clear about the birth you dream.
2. Look at all your internal stuff – fears, tensions, issues, guilt, secrets…
3. Now let go in all the varied ways outlined in this book.
4. Focus on the light of your dream, BE the light of your dream as if it is true for you right now.
5. Focus on the Goddess energy as well as your own divinity: imagine the Goddess in front of you and become her.
6. Relax and trust in your heart, and follow the energy whilst doing whatever emotional clearing you may need to do.
7. Remember that your daily practise is not "work" but a joyous time of filling with light, tuning in and connecting with yourself and your baby!

7 Key Pointers for Creating Good Vibrations in the Aquarian Age

1. Thoughts = reality
2. All is a mirror for what is going on within, keep removing the blocks and shadows
3. Bless All
4. JAPA - Chanting God's name
5. MANTRA - Chanting the words of God
6. AFFIRM - all your words are affirmations, remember your beauty and worth with all your thoughts and emotions
7. TUNE IN and only FOLLOW THE LIGHT and your INTUITION at all times

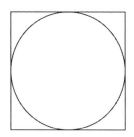

A Birthing Message from the Divine Mother

"Go then, beautiful woman, Divine Mother, to birth.

And birth knowing all is well and all will be well for you.

You are blessed, your baby is blessed, your birth is blessed.
And know that wherever you are and whatever you do, your birth is an absolutely sacred and important event since you are birthing a child of God into this world of form.
As you sit here with your beautiful belly glowing with life, know that you are deeply connected to God as Goddess bringing forth Life onto Earth.
You are in the fullness of your power right now.
You are a channel for Spirit and for Life.
You are a Child of God birthing into the world another Being, another Child of God; and as such you matter most to us dear one, you matter beyond life since you are deeply blessed with a love so profound that you could not even imagine it.
You are surrendering your body for humankind at a very deep level and, as such, Goddess blesses you beyond words and beyond comparisons.

Birth well, dear one.

Know that you are deeply blessed and that all is as it should be.

Blessings, Glorious Woman. Please know how important you are, wherever and whoever you may be.

So be it and so it is for the highest good of all concerned.

Amen."

"A starchild rides the crest of light, and bathed in light, is born in love, rejoicing!"

The Return of Bird Tribes by Ken Carey

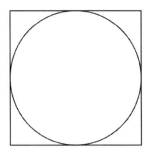

Appendix

Supporting Evidence for the Success of Intuitive Birth Techniques

There are many people who have researched the impact of sacred and holistic birthing on children.

This research work examines things such as - how relaxation creates easy birthing; how home births and sacred births create more emotionally advanced babies; the long lasting effects on the child and mother of a traumatic birth etc Postnatal effects from a traumatic birth can include: feeding problems for either/both mother or/and child, jaundice, colic, depression, sibling rivalry, emotional disturbances in the child and impaired intelligence. Health carers taking the baby away from the mother straight after birth can automatically set up a distance, which in some cases has led to issues such as postnatal depression, breastfeeding problems etc.

Just a few examples of the recent investigative work follow:

Joseph Clinton Pearce clearly analyses exactly why and how the child who is gently birthed and bonded with his/her mother is shown to be highly advanced, in his book *Magical Child*. For example, his research work in Uganda shows how, at 2 days of age *"these infants sat bolt upright, held only by the forearms... and they smiled and smiled"*. He analyses the many ways that these Ugandan babies were highly advanced in his chapter "breaking the bond" . He writes of the *"1956 studies by Marcelle Geber in Kenya and Uganda ... finding most advanced infants ever observed anywhere. They were born in the home, generally delivered by the mother herself. The child was never separated from the mother, who massaged, caressed, sang to, and fondled her infant continually. The mother carried her unswaddled infant in a sling, next to her bare breast, continually. She slept with her infant. The infant fed continuously, according to its own schedule. These infants were awake a surprising amount of time – alert, watchful, happy, calm. They virtually never cried. Their mothers were bonded to them and sensed their every need before that need had to be expressed by crying.....".*

He goes on to cite examples of the damage done in hospital births throughout his book, for example *"Frederick LeBoyer, a conventional French obstetrician who delivered 9,000 babies by standard methods, noticed that France had over 1 million dysfunctional children.... he realised that hospital deliveries were damaging the infants"*. He also goes on to state that the highly advanced babies in Uganda were totally abandoned by their mother at 4 years of age according to strict, unbreakable customs and this abandonment immediately undid all emotional advancement that each infant had conveyed.

Vivette Glover, Professor of Perinatal Psychobiology at Imperial College London, trained as a biochemist at Oxford and did her PhD in neurochemistry at University College London. In 1997, she set up the Fetal and Neonatal Stress Research Group. The aims are to study fetal and neonatal stress responses, methods to reduce them and their long term effects. The effects of psychopathology in the mother, both on the developing fetus and longer term on the child are also being studied. This is a new field for study, and one which involves linking obstetrics, paediatrics, psychology and psychiatry. Recent projects of interest include studies characterising the stress responses of the fetus and the first trial of analgesia in the fetus; studies showing that maternal antenatal stress or anxiety increases the risk for a range of emotional, behavioural and cognitive adverse outcomes for the child; and studies showing possible mechanisms by which maternal stress or anxiety may affect the development of the fetus. This work is demonstrating the importance of the fetal period and the emotional state of the mother during pregnancy on the later neurodevelopment of the child. Glover has published over 400 papers.

In "The Secret Life of the Unborn Child", Dr. Thomas Verny and John Kelly analyse and discuss the importance of the mother's bonding with the baby for emotional harmony, leading to a happy and advanced baby. They spent two decades researching the earliest stages of life: "*At sixteen weeks the unborn child shies away from light. At twenty weeks there is a response to speech patterns. At twenty five weeks the baby can kick in time to music. And at six months the unborn baby can understand the subtle shifts of its mother's emotions.*"

Simon House, who holds a Cambridge degree is in Natural Sciences and Theology, spent eight years marketing in a pharmaceutical, food and agrochemical company. Conviction that health could not be found in a bottle led to 30 years as an Anglican parish priest. House focuses on the effects of environmental changes on human brain development, clarified through the perspective of evolution, of marine life as well as terrestrial life, and now of epigenetics. These aspects throw light on finer ways of parenting to protect the brain from adverse changes in the nurturing environment, and from ecological changes caused by the power of the human brain itself to change the biosphere. This critical interaction between brain and environment can be ameliorated by skilful management. He is passionate about integrating these insights so that professionals and the public engage in reclaiming primal and ecological health, and so generate children healthy in body and mind. For 10 years he has been presenting an integral view to international congresses.

In 2006, House updated Roy Ridgway's book 'The Unborn Child', drawing profoundly on Lake, Liedloff, Odent and many psychotherapists, including his own experience. He also added a new section, on the effects of nutrition prior to conception on brain development, drawing on the outstanding brain chemistry of Professor Michael Crawford and others, whose research he had reviewed in *Generating Healthy People: Stages in reproduction particularly vulnerable to xenobiotic hazards and nutritional deficits* (Medline). In *Generating Healthy Brains*, a cutting-edge conference in London 2006, House brought together the leaders of the International Society for Prenatal and Perinatal Psychiatry and Medicine (ISPPM) and the McCarrison Society for Nutrition and Health. Speakers' articles also are on Medline, including his own, Nurturing the brain, nutritionally and emotionally, from before conception to late adolescence (2007). At the recent ISPPM Congress he received the Elda Scarzella Mazzochi Award for his contribution to shalom/salaam – to health, completeness, peacefulness.

His publications include
1.   Nurturing the brain, nutritionally and emotionally, from before conception to late adolescence. In *Generating Healthy Brains* (2007). Nutrition and Health 19.1-2. (Find: house nurturing brain)
2.   *The Unborn Child: beginning a whole life and overcoming problems of early origin.* Ridgway & House (2006). Karnac Books
3.   Generating Healthy People: Stages in reproduction particularly vulnerable to xenobiotic hazards and nutritional deficits. (2000). *Nutrition and Health* 14.3
4.   Primal Integration Therapy – School of Dr Frank Lake MB, MRC Psych, DPM, JSPPM (1999); JOPPPAH (2000).
5.   *The Struggle for Wholeness in People and in the World*, S George's House, Windsor Castle (1978)

For several decades, **Michel Odent** has been instrumental in influencing the history of childbirth and health research. As a practitioner, he developed the maternity unit at Pithiviers Hospital in France in the 1960s and 70s. He is familiarly known as the obstetrician who introduced the concept of birthing pools and home-like birthing rooms. His approach has been featured in eminent medical journals such as The Lancet, and in TV documentaries such as the BBC film *Birth Reborn*. With six midwives, he was in charge of about one thousand births a year and achieved ideal statistics with low rates of intervention. After his hospital career he practiced home birth.

As a researcher he founded the Primal Health Research Centre in London (UK), which focuses upon the long-term consequences of early experiences. An overview of the Primal Health Research data bank clearly indicates that health is to a great extent shaped during the primal period (from conception until the first birthday). It also suggests that the way we are born has long-term consequences in terms of sociability and aggressiveness or, otherwise speaking, capacity to love.

Author of approximately 50 scientific papers, Odent has written 11 books, which have been published in 21 languages. In his books he developed the art of turning traditional questions around, looking at the question of "how to develop good health" rather than at that of "how to prevent disease", and at the question of "how the capacity to love develops", rather than at that of "how to prevent violence". His books include *The Scientification of Love* (1999) and *The Farmer and the Obstetrician* (2002) and they raise urgent questions about the future of our civilization. His latest book, *Childbirth in the Age of Plastics* was published in 2011.

Birth into being (www.birthintobeing.com) is a movement set up by a Russian woman named **Elena Tonetti** and this has formed the base of many new age birth movements such as Ecstatic Birth. It is also based on the fact that to birth well we need to eliminate fears and tensions:

"The quality of our civilization largely depends on the way we procreate. The way we arrive into this world defines our capacity for love, compassion, intimacy. Conscious conception and birth are an integral part of conscious living. When parents create a new baby in full awareness of the effect their actions and thoughts have on their unborn child, humankind

is given another chance to thrive. The quality of our life is defined, first of all, by the quality of attention and love received while we are still in our mother's womb! Secondly, the life is defined by the quality of our birth itself. There is an overwhelming body of evidence that birth trauma is responsible for addictions, violence, low self-esteem, poor problem-solving skills, short attention span and a host of physical health problems…

Non-traumatized babies, who are conceived and born in Love, display an amazing degree of intelligence, kindness, common sense and good health. As they grow they prove themselves to be good communicators, peaceful, caring, alert, self-motivated human beings. Natural birth does require some preparation nowadays, for attention to the art of birthing has been in decline for many generations. In tribal life it was supposed to be a mother's gift to her daughter, a natural obvious transmission. But with the modern day stress level and easy access to drugs, in the US 95% of births are considered traumatic. 50% rated as moderate trauma, 45% of them are rated as severely traumatic. Our species has an amazing built-in mechanism for procreation. Our bodies are designed to reproduce naturally, with grace and ease. To be able to relax in a bath tub during labor was found extremely helpful by millions of women. However, waterbirth by itself does not guarantee the degree of consciousness, of non-trauma, that we desire and deserve. We, as spiritual beings, have the capacity to experience the transformative power of birth that connects us with deeper understanding of life. When a new human being that did not exist before, enters into our world, the veil separating our reality from the Great Unseen becomes very transparent for a short period of time. This gives us an opportunity to experience, first hand, the ecstatic bliss of ONENESS with all, a state in which separation does not exist, where Love prevails. When Love is an integral part of the birthing field, a woman has access to the power of creation that is working through her. The more power there is in her field the less force she will need to use, because Love is a highly coherent field. And vice versa: the less power she has, the more force it would require to deliver a baby. In the beginning every one of us was a tiny infant - speechless, vulnerable, in desperate need of love and care. In our soft, warm hands we are holding the keys to the thriving of our species! We have the capacity to enhance the quality of life in one generation through bringing our loving, conscious awareness into our people-making practices. Birth is a powerful initiation, a rite of passage for all involved, which enables us to create a beautiful Life on this planet. It is our birthright!"

Dr Bruce H. Lipton is a cellular and developmental biologist who has discovered a new science that reveals the mechanism by which the beliefs and emotions of parents influence the selection and even rewriting of their children's genetic code. *"Parental "programming" is first initiated in the formation of the germ cells (eggs and sperm) through a process called "genomic imprinting". The parents' influence in shaping the life of their child are further extended in the watery world of the womb when the prenatal brain begins to acquire environmental experiences. Subsequently the character and potential of a child can be profoundly nurtured or damaged through birth bonding and parenting skills."*

The obstetrician Dr Grantly Dick-Read attended a birth in 1913 that changed his life. He attended a birth in the slums of London where a girl refused to take chloroform. With little more than gentle breathing, she birthed her baby. When he asked why she had refused the chloroform, she replied, "It didn't hurt. It wasn't meant to, was it, doctor?"

This question lead Dick Read to compare this birth with the so called "usual" births which were associated with terror and agony. He then experienced another birthing woman whilst in the trenches during World War One. She seemed oblivious to the war around her, easily birthed her baby, wrapped it up and went on her way. In Africa, again he saw a birthing woman easily birth against a hedge. Dick Read started to realise that the easy births he had been witnessing were all lacking one important thing – lacking fear. Further study led him to the understanding that fear in birth causes the arteries to the uterus to constrict and become tense. This causes pain. If a woman is relaxed then the cervix can naturally thin out, relaxant hormones (since named 'endorphins') can be released into her body, and her body can pulsate and release the baby well. Dick-Read called this understanding the "Fear-tension-pain cycle". His colleagues refused to believe that birth could be pain free, and people still believe this today. His theories were printed in the 1950s in a book called "Revelations in Childbirth", known in the USA as "Childbirth Without Fear".

Bibliography of quotations referred to in this Book

The Seven Spiritual Laws of Success by Deepak Chopra
The Tibetan Book of the Dead
Ponder on This by Alice A. Bailey
A Course in Miracles by the Foundation for Inner Peace
The Bhagavad Gita
Tao Te Ching
Katha Upanishad I
Birth without Doctors: Conversations with Traditional Midwives by Jacqueline Vincent Priya
Anything Can Be Healed by Martin Brofman
The Way of the Sun by White Eagle.
The Diamond Light by Violet Starre
The Power of The Magdalene by Stuart Wilson and Joanna Prentis
Ina May's Guide to Childbirth by Ina May Gaskin
The Power of Now by Eckhart Tolle
The Complete Ascension Manual: How to Achieve Ascension in This Lifetime by Joshua Stone
Ascended Masters Light the Way: Beacons of Ascension by Joshua Stone
Huna: Ancient Secrets for Modern Living by Serge Kahili King
Love without Conditions by Paul Ferrini
Ancient Futures: Learning from Ladakh by Helena Norberg Hodge
Paths to God, Living the Bhagavad Gita by Ram Dass
Be Here Now by Ram Dass
The Gentle Birth Method: The Month-by-month Jeyarani Way Programme by Gowri Motha
Marsden Wagener M.D.
Love You Deserve: A Spiritual Guide to Genuine Love by Scott and Shannon Peck
A Book of Angels by Sophy Burnham
Buddhism for Mothers: A Calm Approach to Caring for Yourself and Your Children by Sarah
Napthali
Mothering and Fathering: The Gender difference in Child Rearing by Thine Thevenin
Empowerment and Integration Through The Goddess by Rev. Wistancia Stone and Dr Joshua
David Stone.
Ramana Maharashi
Non Violent Communication by Marshall B. Rosenberg
The Secret Life of the Unborn Child by Dr Thomas Verny with John Kelly.
GeorGina Kelly, G. (2004) Birthing and Saying the Great Yes. The Mother Magazine. Autumn,
Issue 11.
The Red Tent by Anita Diamant
Birthing from Within by Pam England
Holistic Herbal for Mother and Baby by Kitty Champion
Jacqueline Vincent Priya.
You are Your Child's First Teacher by Rahima Bladwin Dancy
Joseph Chilton Pearce
Living in the Light by Shakti Gawain
The Return of Bird Tribes by Ken Carey
Magical Child by Joseph Chilton Pearce
Val J Taylor, midwife Sussex
"Man to Man, The Men's Teachings Of Yogi Bhajan" by Yogi Bahaman
I Am a Woman: Creative, Sacred & Invincible--Essential Kriyas For Women In The Aquarian Age
by Yogi Bhajan
The Aquarian Teacher by Yogi Bhajan
Journey Of Souls:Case Studies of Life Between Lives, by Ph.D. Michael Newton
www.rawmomsummit.com
www.informedparent.co.uk

Disclaimer

All information presented in this book comes from the personal beliefs of the author, and is not presented as medical advise. Acceptance or otherwise of the validity of the methods and information presented in this book, is a matter of personal belief & no claim is made as to the accuracy of information provided. Therefore the reader is advised to use their own judgment as to whether to act on the basis of information provided. All exercises carried out are done so are the reader's responsibility and carried out at the reader's own risk. The author claims no responsibility for any situation caused from the information provided. It is advised that before carrying out any exercise or herbal treatment mentioned, that you seek health care advise.

Ishtara Rose

Ishtara Rose is a born sensitive. After discovering Reiki in 1993 following some profound awakening spiritual experiences, she went onto study Angelic Healing, Shiatsu, Past Life Regression, Indian Head Massage, the Body - Mirror system, as well as joining various mystery schools, alongside a career in the arts.

When Ishtara became pregnant in 2006 she went on a mission to prepare for a natural and healthy birth using the meditation and holistic techniques that she had always been passionate about and practised. In preparing for birth, Ishtara brought her knowledge together to create a unique journey which included diving into Meditation, Mantra and Visualisation techniques as well as enjoying looking into many topics from Nutrition, Acupuncture, Herbal medicine, Aryuveda, Energy Healing, Yoga (Hatha and Kundalini), Massage, Reflexology, Cranial Sacral methods, Shamanism, Naturopathy, Homeopathy, Angel Visualisation, Spiritual Healing, Shamanic Journeying, Hypnosis...to name but a few.

When Ishtara became pregnant again the following year, she was naturally able to further integrate these methods for birthing. During this inner journey towards her next birth, she birthed a new self, becoming also a light channel for birthing messages that came through in meditations.

During these special times, Ishtara had what she now calls Rose Awakening, when the Marys came to commune with her and expand her mediumship. As she started to write the messages down she felt inspired to gather the material together into a book to share both the birthing methods and meditations to help empower other women to also create and journey through their own beautiful and sacred pregnancy and birth initiations of their most sacred and divine and unique inner rose.

Ishtara went onto to become a Kundalini Yoga teacher then later trained as a Priestess and then High Priestess where she expanded her mediumship further, through several years of initiations taking place in the hills of UK, Italy and France. She finally launched Way of the Rose in 2017 after a message from Mary Magdalene to do so.

Since 2017, Ishtara has run various Magdalene Rose Priestess Temples as a teacher, medium, channel and rose activator whilst also sharing Mediumship Advancement courses, Light Transmission audios and Healing Packages, including her channelled Rose Reiki Healing ray. You can find all her latest audios and courses online at www.wayoftherose.co.uk or follow her on social media.

This book is a revised edition 2022 from the original material that was initially written in and around 2009 and self published in 2013.

Other books by Ishtara Rose include Mary Magdalene, Way of the Rose.

www.wayoftherose.co.uk

Printed in Great Britain
by Amazon

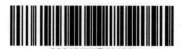